T0348631

Pregnancy and Endocrine Disorders

Editor

MARK E. MOLITCH

ENDOCRINOLOGY AND METABOLISM CLINICS OF NORTH AMERICA

www.endo.theclinics.com

Consulting Editor
ADRIANA G. IOACHIMESCU

September 2019 • Volume 48 • Number 3

ELSEVIER

1600 John F. Kennedy Boulevard • Suite 1800 • Philadelphia, Pennsylvania, 19103-2899

http://www.theclinics.com

ENDOCRINOLOGY AND METABOLISM CLINICS OF NORTH AMERICA Volume 48, Number 3
September 2019 ISSN 0889-8529, ISBN 13: 978-0-323-68224-4

Editor: Stacy Eastman
Developmental Editor: Casey Potter

Endocrinology and Metabolism Clinics of North America (ISSN 0889-8529) is published quarterly by Elsevier Inc., 360 Park Avenue South, New York, NY 10010-1710. Months of issue are March, June, September, and December. Periodicals postage paid at New York, NY and additional mailing offices. Subscription prices are USD 371.00 per year for US individuals, USD 761.00 per year for US institutions, USD 100.00 per year for US students and residents, USD 454.00 per year for Canadian individuals, USD 941.00 per year for Canadian institutions, USD 497.00 per year for international individuals, USD 941.00 per year for international institutions, and USD 245.00 per year for international and Canadian and foreign students/residents. To receive student/resident rate, orders must be accompanied by name of affiliated institution, date of term, and the signature of program/ residency coordinator on institution letterhead. Orders will be billed at individual rate until proof of status is received. Foreign air speed delivery is included in all *Clinics* subscription prices. All prices are subject to change without notice. **POSTMASTER:** Send address changes to *Endocrinology and Metabolism Clinics of North America*, Elsevier Health Sciences Division, Subscription Customer Service, 3251 Riverport Lane, Maryland Heights, MO 63043. **Customer Service: Telephone: 1-800-654-2452** (U.S. and Canada); **1-314-447-8871** (outside U.S. and Canada). **Fax: 1-314-447-8029. E-mail: journalscustomerservice-usa@elsevier.com (for print support); journalsonlinesupport-usa@elsevier.com (for online support)**.

Reprints. For copies of 100 or more, of articles in this publication, please contact the Commercial Rights Department, Elsevier Inc., 360 Park Avenue South, New York, NY 10010-1710; phone: +1-212-633-3874; fax: +1-212-633-3820; E-mail: reprints@elsevier.com.

Endocrinology and Metabolism Clinics of North America is covered in *MEDLINE/PubMed (Index Medicus)*, *EMBASE/Excerpta Medica, Current Contents/Clinical Medicine, Current Contents/Life Sciences, Science Citation Index, ISI/BIOMED, BIOSIS,* and *Chemical Abstracts*.

Contributors

CONSULTING EDITOR

ADRIANA G. IOACHIMESCU, MD, PhD
Professor of Medicine (Endocrinology) and Neurosurgery, Emory University School of Medicine, Atlanta, Georgia, USA

EDITOR

MARK E. MOLITCH, MD
Martha Leland Sherwin Professor of Endocrinology, Division of Endocrinology, Metabolism and Molecular Medicine, Department of Medicine, Northwestern University Feinberg School of Medicine, Chicago, Illinois, USA

AUTHORS

ERIK K. ALEXANDER, MD
Professor of Medicine, The Thyroid Section, Division of Endocrinology, Diabetes, and Hypertension, Brigham and Women's Hospital, Harvard Medical School, Boston, Massachusetts, USA

TREVOR E. ANGELL, MD
Assistant Professor of Clinical Medicine, Division of Endocrinology and Diabetes, Keck School of Medicine of USC, Los Angeles, California, USA

CLAIRE CASEY, PhD
Regional Centre for Endocrinology and Diabetes, Royal Victoria Hospital, Belfast, Northern Ireland, United Kingdom

PHILIPPE CHANSON, MD
Assistance Publique-Hôpitaux de Paris (P.C.), Hôpitaux Universitaires Paris-Sud, Hôpital de Bicêtre, Service d'Endocrinologie et des Maladies de la Reproduction, Centre de Référence des Maladies Rares de l'Hypophyse, UMR S-1185, Fac Med Paris Sud, Université Paris-Saclay, Le Kremlin-Bicêtre, France

GRAEME EISENHOFER, PhD
Department of Medicine III, Carl Gustav Carus University Medical Centre, Institute of Clinical Chemistry and Laboratory Medicine, Medical Faculty Carl Gustav Carus, Technische Universität Dresden, Dresden, Germany

MOSHE HOD, MD
FIGO Pregnancy and NCD Committee, Professor, Department of Obstetrics and Gynecology, Chief Consultant in Perinatal Medicine, Clalit Health Services, Mor Women's Health Center, Rabin Medical Center, Tel Aviv University, Tel Aviv, Israel

WENYU HUANG, MD, PhD
Assistant Professor of Medicine, Division of Endocrinology, Metabolism and Molecular Medicine, Northwestern University Feinberg School of Medicine, Chicago, Illinois, USA

JAMI L. JOSEFSON, MD, MS
Associate Professor, Division of Endocrinology, Department of Pediatrics, Northwestern University Feinberg School of Medicine, Ann and Robert H. Lurie Children's Hospital of Chicago, Chicago, Illinois, USA

ANIL KAPUR, MD
Chairman, World Diabetes Foundation, Bagsverd, Denmark; FIGO Pregnancy and NCD Committee, Petah Tiqwa, Israel

KRISTEN KOBALY, MD
Assistant Professor of Clinical Medicine, Division of Endocrinology, Diabetes and Metabolism, Perelman School of Medicine, University of Pennsylvania, Perelman Center for Advanced Medicine, Philadelphia, Pennsylvania, USA

JOHAN F. LANGENHUIJSEN, MD, PhD
Department of Urology, Radboud University Medical Centre, Nijmegen, The Netherlands

KATHARINA LANGTON, MSc
Institute of Clinical Chemistry and Laboratory Medicine, Medical Faculty Carl Gustav Carus, Technische Universität Dresden, Dresden, Germany

JOHN H. LAZARUS, MD
Thyroid Research Group, Systems Immunity Research Institute, Cardiff University School of Medicine, UHW, Cardiff, United Kingdom

JULIUS SIMONI LEERE, MD
Clinical Assistant, PhD Student, Department of Clinical Medicine and Endocrinology, Aalborg University, Department of Endocrinology, Aalborg University Hospital, Aalborg, Denmark

JACQUES W.M. LENDERS, MD, PhD
Department of Internal Medicine, Radboud University Medical Centre, Nijmegen, The Netherlands; Department of Medicine III, Carl Gustav Carus University Medical Centre, Dresden, Germany

SUSAN J. MANDEL, MD, MPH
Director, Clinical Endocrinology and Diabetes, University of Pennsylvania Health System, Professor of Medicine and Radiology, Division of Endocrinology, Diabetes and Metabolism, Perelman School of Medicine, University of Pennsylvania, Perelman Center for Advanced Medicine, Philadelphia, Pennsylvania, USA

DAVID R. McCANCE, MD
Regional Centre for Endocrinology and Diabetes, Royal Victoria Hospital, Belfast, Northern Ireland, United Kingdom

HAROLD DAVID McINTYRE, MD, FRACP
FIGO Pregnancy and NCD Committee, UQ Mater Clinical Unit, Professor, Faculty of Medicine, Director of Obstetric Medicine, Mater Health Services, University of Queensland, Raymond Terrace, South Brisbane, Queensland, Australia

BOYD E. METZGER, MD
Emeritus Professor of Medicine, Division of Endocrinology, Metabolism and Molecular Medicine, Department of Medicine, Northwestern University Feinberg School of Medicine, Chicago, Illinois, USA

MARK E. MOLITCH, MD
Martha Leland Sherwin Professor of Endocrinology, Division of Endocrinology, Metabolism and Molecular Medicine, Department of Medicine, Northwestern University Feinberg School of Medicine, Chicago, Illinois, USA

NICOLE REISCH, MD
Medizinische Klinik IV, Department of Endocrinology, Klinikum der Universität München, München, Germany

EMILY D. SZMUILOWICZ, MD, MS
Associate Professor, Department of Medicine, Division of Endocrinology, Metabolism and Molecular Medicine, Northwestern University Feinberg School of Medicine, Chicago, Illinois, USA

PETER N. TAYLOR, PhD
Thyroid Research Group, Systems Immunity Research Institute, Cardiff University School of Medicine, UHW, Cardiff, United Kingdom

PETER VESTERGAARD, MD, PhD, DMSc
Department of Endocrinology, Aalborg University Hospital, Professor, Head of Research, Steno Diabetes Center North Jutland, Aalborg, Denmark

Contents

Although it has been accepted for decades that women with gestational diabetes mellitus (GDM) are at high risk for future development of type 2 diabetes, vigorous debate regarding the value of detecting and treating GDM has persisted into the twenty-first century. Although results from 2 randomized trials provide strong evidence that treating GDM reduces adverse perinatal outcomes, it remains to be determined whether treatment impacts long-term offspring outcomes. Insulin is the first-line pharmacologic treatment and is added when glycemic goals are not met with nutritional modifications. Oral agent use is controversial, as data on long-term offspring outcomes are lacking.

Congenital malformations and perinatal mortality rates remain severalfold higher in pregnant women with type 1 diabetes than in the background population, and still only a minority of women plan their pregnancy. Optimizing glycemic control is the accepted goal, but remains challenging, and must be constantly balanced against the risks of hypoglycemia. Recent advances including Continuous Glucose Monitoring Systems, Continuous Subcutaneous Insulin Infusion, Closed Loop Devices and very Fast Acting Insulin Aspart analogs offer new possibilities to increase glucose time in target in selected, motivated patients, however their relative roles and indication for use require further elucidation. The importance of education cannot be overstated.

Hyperglycemia is common during pregnancy, involving multisystem adaptations. Pregnancy-induced metabolic changes increase insulin resistance. Pregnancy-induced insulin resistance adds to preexisting insulin resistance. Preexisting pancreatic β-cell defect compromises the ability to enhance insulin secretion, leading to hyperglycemia. Women with type 2 DM have similar rates of major congenital malformations, stillbirth, and neonatal mortality, but an even higher risk of perinatal mortality. In utero type 2 DM exposure confers greater risk and reduces time to development of type 2 DM in offspring. Preconception care to improve metabolic control in women with type 2 diabetes is critical.

Clinical hyperthyroidism affects 0.1% to 0.4% of pregnancies. Gestational thyrotoxicosis is due to homology of the structure of TSH and HCG, which weakly stimulates the TSH receptor. Graves' disease (GD) most commonly causes clinically significant hyperthyroidism. Given concerns for teratogenicity from antithyroid drugs, these may be discontinued in low-risk GD patients. High-risk patients are treated with propylthiouracil in the first trimester then may transition to methimazole. Surgery is reserved for special circumstances; radioactive iodine is contraindicated. In late pregnancy, GD may remit; postpartum relapse is common. Measurement of serum thyrotropin receptor antibodies identifies pregnancies at-risk for fetal and neonatal hyperthyroidism.

Thyroid hormone is essential for pregnancy and ensuring fetal development. Pregnancy also places substantial demands on the thyroid axis. Overt hypothyroidism is associated with substantial adverse obstetric and offspring outcomes and requires treatment. Borderline thyroid dysfunction is common in women and associated with adverse obstetric and offspring outcomes, although benefits of screening for and treating borderline thyroid function are unclear. Many women are established on thyroid hormone replacement before pregnancy and doses need increasing during pregnancy. Care is taken to prevent overreplacement. Universal thyroid screening in pregnancy is being undertaken in several countries, although it remains a matter of debate.

Thyroid nodules and thyroid cancer are common conditions and may be identified during pregnancy. The comprehensive evaluation of thyroid nodules during pregnancy includes a medical history, physical examination, ultrasound assessment, and (when indicated) an ultrasound-guided fine-needle aspiration biopsy. Most thyroid cancers detected during pregnancy will not grow nor pose significant risk during gestation, and thyroid surgery in pregnant women poses higher risks than in nonpregnant women. Through a balanced and informed approach to the clinical care of this unique population, outcomes can be optimized for both the mother and the fetus.

Pituitary adenomas are common. The impact of pituitary tumors on fertility are mainly caused by oversecretion and/or undersecretion of pituitary hormones or compression of pituitary stalk and normal pituitary tissue by the tumor. Diagnosing and managing pituitary tumors during pregnancy involve many challenges, including the effect of hormone excess or deficiency on pregnancy outcome, changes in the pituitary or pituitary-related hormones, changes in tumor size, and the impact of various treatments of pituitary tumors on maternal and fetal outcomes. This article discusses the diagnosis and treatment of patients with prolactinomas, acromegaly, Cushing disease, and other pituitary tumors during pregnancy.

Philippe Chanson

Diagnosis of lymphocytic hypophysitis occurring in the peripartum period is based on clinical and neuroradiological data and does not require a biopsy. Its course is generally spontaneously favorable in terms of mass effect but may require the administration of corticosteroids or even transsphenoidal resection. The course of pituitary deficiencies is highly variable; some cases recover over time, whereas others persist indefinitely. Sheehan syndrome is very rare in developed countries. Because agalactia and amenorrhea are often neglected, the diagnosis is generally delayed. Diabetes insipidus occurring in late pregnancy is caused by the increased placental production of vasopressinase and disappears after delivery.

Jacques W.M. Lenders, Katharina Langton, Johan F. Langenhuijsen, and Graeme Eisenhofer

Pheochromocytoma during pregnancy, although rare, is a perilous condition. The wellbeing of mother and fetus are at stake if not diagnosed and treated antenatally and timely. The diagnosis is frequently overlooked because of the aspecific nature of signs and symptoms and confusion with pregnancy-related hypertension. Measurements of plasma or urinary free metanephrines have the highest diagnostic accuracy. MRI is preferred over ultrasonography. The optimal time for surgical removal is before 24 weeks of gestation or at/after delivery. Laparoscopic adrenalectomy should be preceded by medical pretreatment. Cesarean delivery is preferred in these patients; vaginal delivery might be considered in selected pretreated patients.

Nicole Reisch

Fertility rates in classic congenital adrenal hyperplasia caused by 21-hydroxylase deficiency are substantially decreased for various reasons, including hormonal, anatomic, psychosocial, and psychosexual causes. However, fecundity is comparable with the general population. Under optimal hormone replacement, the course and outcome of pregnancies is also good. This article summarizes successful gestational management, including preconceptional considerations, adjustment of hormone replacement during pregnancy, delivery and lactation, as well as the prevention of adrenal crises. In nonclassic 21-hydroxylase deficiency, preconceptional low-dose hydrocortisone replacement normalizes the otherwise increased miscarriage rate. Pregnancy reports in rarer forms of congenital adrenal hyperplasia are summarized as well.

Physiologic changes during pregnancy include calcium, phosphate, and calciotropic hormone status. Calcium metabolic disorders are rare in pregnancy and management with close calcium and vitamin D control and supplementation. Primary hyperparathyroidism is mostly asymptomatic and does not affect conception or pregnancy. It requires control of plasma calcium levels. Surgical intervention may be indicated. Data on severe cases are missing. Osteoporosis in or before pregnancy is rare but usually diagnosed from fractures. Medical treatment other than supplementation is contraindicated. Vitamin D deficiency is common and may affect conception and increase complications. Current evidence does not prove vitamin D supplements effective in improving outcomes.

ENDOCRINOLOGY AND METABOLISM CLINICS OF NORTH AMERICA

SERIES OF RELATED INTEREST

Medical Clinics
https://www.medical.theclinics.com

VISIT THE CLINICS ONLINE!
Access your subscription at:
www.theclinics.com

Foreword

Pregnancy and Endocrine Disorders

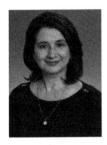

Adriana G. Ioachimescu, MD, PhD
Consulting Editor

It is my great pleasure to introduce the "Pregnancy and Endocrine Disorders" issue of the *Endocrinology and Metabolism Clinics of North America*. The guest editor is Dr Mark E. Molitch, Professor of Endocrinology, Metabolism, and Molecular Medicine at the Northwestern University Feinberg School of Medicine in Chicago.

The intersection between endocrine diseases and pregnancy can influence both maternal and fetal outcomes. In patients with preexisting endocrine conditions, like diabetes mellitus, hypothyroidism, Graves disease, or pituitary tumors, preconception counseling and care are of paramount importance. In patients who experience de novo endocrine abnormalities during pregnancy, making a correct diagnosis can be challenging and requires a thorough understanding of the physiologic hormone changes during pregnancy. Biochemical testing should be interpreted with caution to account for alterations in binding globulins, placental hormone secretion, and other factors. Furthermore, diagnosis can be challenging because some imaging tests are not safe to use during pregnancy. Once the diagnosis is made, management is complex due to potential teratogenicity of drugs used (eg, antithyroid or cortisol-lowering medications), placental transfer of drugs, and risks associated with surgery. The key to success is a multidisciplinary collaboration between endocrinologists, obstetricians, neonatologists, and other specialists with experience in their field.

The guest editor dedicated several articles to the different facets of hyperglycemia in pregnancy. The articles nicely summarize the currently recommended glucose thresholds and targets and medical therapy considerations for types 1, 2, and gestational diabetes as well as studies related to how pregnancy outcomes are affected by glucose control. Thyroid function abnormalities and thyroid nodules are also encountered in many pregnant women. The authors address the debate regarding universal versus targeted screening for thyroid disease in pregnancy as well as outcomes expected from correction of borderline thyroid test abnormalities.

Endocrinol Metab Clin N Am 48 (2019) xiii–xiv
https://doi.org/10.1016/j.ecl.2019.06.002
0889-8529/19/© 2019 Published by Elsevier Inc.

endo.theclinics.com

Pheochromocytomas and paraganglioma are rare but have potential devastating consequences in pregnancy, when medical and surgical treatment entail several caveats. Patients with pituitary tumors also require special attention during pregnancy because some patients with macroadenomas are at risk for mass effect symptoms, and other patients carry a higher risk of metabolic and cardiovascular complications from hormone hypersecretion. Nontumor pituitary gland pathology can also occur during pregnancy or after delivery, including lymphocytic hypophysitis and Sheehan syndrome.

Patients with congenital adrenal hyperplasia have an increased risk of infertility and pregnancy complications compared with the general population. The authors nicely summarize preconceptional care and adjustment of hormone replacement during pregnancy, delivery, and lactation.

Calcium and phosphate metabolism undergo changes during pregnancy that are well described in a dedicated article in this issue. With the exception of vitamin D deficiency, calcium metabolic disorders and osteoporosis are rarely encountered; however, management of such conditions during pregnancy can be challenging.

I hope you will find this issue of the *Endocrinology and Metabolism Clinics of North America* informative and helpful in your practice. I thank Dr Molitch for guest-editing this important collection of articles and the authors for their excellent contributions. I also would like to acknowledge the Elsevier editorial staff for their support.

Adriana G. Ioachimescu, MD, PhD
Emory University School of Medicine
1365 B Clifton Rd, Northeast, B6209
Atlanta, GA 30322, USA

E-mail address:
aioachi@emory.edu

Preface

Pregnancy and Endocrine Disorders

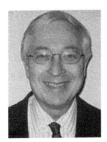

Mark E. Molitch, MD
Editor

Fertility can be affected by a number of endocrine conditions, and treatments with normalization of hormone levels are usually necessary to allow pregnancy to occur. The treatments may then need modification because of potential adverse effects on a developing fetus. For example, the choice of antithyroid agents may need to be altered when pregnancy is anticipated. Another example is what should be done with dopamine agonists or somatostatin analogues in patients with prolactinomas or acromegaly once pregnancy is diagnosed.

Pregnancy itself alters normal physiology and endocrine conditions in a number of ways as a result of a variety of factors. Pregnancy results in an expansion of plasma and red blood cell volume with an increase in glomerular filtration rate, resulting in changes in the normal values for various hormones as well as an increase in the clearance of many of the medications used. Hormone production by the placenta may have profound effects, especially the more than 100-fold rise in estrogen levels, again altering hormone levels and also having direct effects on the pituitary. Placental estrogen, progesterone, lactogen, and possibly the growth hormone variant also function as counterregulatory hormones with respect to insulin and cause insulin resistance and accelerated lipolysis. The placenta produces enzymes that may affect normal endocrine function, especially vasopressinase, which can result in the worsening of subclinical diabetes insipidus.

In this issue, we review the most common endocrine conditions that can affect a woman desiring pregnancy with emphasis on the diagnostic and therapeutic challenges facing the clinician. There are separate articles on type 1, type 2, and gestational diabetes, and the last two include controversial topics, such as the use of oral agents and the new Hyperglycemia and Adverse Pregnancy Outcomes (HAPO) data. Articles on thyroid disease, including thyroid cancer, focus on target hormone levels and the need for medication changes during pregnancy. The challenges posed by

Endocrinol Metab Clin N Am 48 (2019) xv–xvi
https://doi.org/10.1016/j.ecl.2019.06.001
0889-8529/19/© 2019 Published by Elsevier Inc.

endo.theclinics.com

the diagnosis and treatment of the various types of pituitary tumors in pregnancy are reviewed. Pheochromocytomas, adrenal insufficiency, and congenital adrenal hyperplasia are addressed in articles on pregnancy and adrenal disease. Calcium disorders in pregnant women are also reviewed.

Things aren't always straightforward in the management of pregnant women with endocrine diseases, and we hope that the reviews here can provide up-to-date guidance when problems occur.

Mark E. Molitch, MD
Division of Endocrinology, Metabolism &
Molecular Medicine
Department of Medicine
Northwestern University
Feinberg School of Medicine
645 North Michigan Avenue
Suite 530
Chicago, IL 60611, USA

E-mail address:
molitch@northwestern.edu

Gestational Diabetes Mellitus

Emily D. Szmuilowicz, MD, MS[a], Jami L. Josefson, MD, MS[b], Boyd E. Metzger, MD[c],*

KEYWORDS

- Gestational diabetes mellitus • Pregnancy • Diagnosis • Offspring • Outcomes
- Treatment

KEY POINTS

- Although it is well established that women with gestational diabetes mellitus (GDM) are at high risk for future development of T2DM, vigorous debate regarding the value of detecting and treating GDM persists.
- The Hyperglycemia and Adverse Pregnancy Outcome (HAPO) study showed that maternal hyperglycemia less severe than that in diabetes mellitus is associated with increased risks of adverse pregnancy outcomes.
- Increased rates of adiposity and disorders of glucose metabolism in peripubertal offspring exposed to GDM have been demonstrated.
- GDM treatment clearly reduces adverse pregnancy outcomes, although the impact of GDM treatment on long-term offspring outcomes remains to be determined.
- Insulin is considered the first-line pharmacologic treatment and is added when glycemic goals are not met with nutritional modifications. Oral agent use is controversial, as data on long-term offspring outcomes are lacking.

DEFINITION, DIAGNOSIS, DETECTION, AND PREVALENCE
Background

The first diagnostic criteria for gestational diabetes mellitus (GDM) were published by O'Sullivan and Mahan 55 years ago.[1] The criteria were developed from results of a 100-g oral glucose tolerance test (OGTT) during pregnancy in an unselected group

Disclosure Statement: None.
a Division of Endocrinology, Metabolism and Molecular Medicine, Department of Medicine, Northwestern University Feinberg School of Medicine, 645 North Michigan Avenue, 530-24, Chicago, IL 60611, USA; b Division of Endocrinology, Department of Pediatrics, Northwestern University Feinberg School of Medicine, Ann and Robert H. Lurie Children's Hospital of Chicago, 225 East Chicago Avenue, Box 54, Chicago, IL 60611, USA; c Division of Endocrinology, Metabolism and Molecular Medicine, Department of Medicine, Northwestern University Feinberg School of Medicine, Tarry Building, Room 12-703, 300 East Superior, Chicago, IL 60611, USA
* Corresponding author.
E-mail address: bem@northwestern.edu

Endocrinol Metab Clin N Am 48 (2019) 479–493
https://doi.org/10.1016/j.ecl.2019.05.001
0889-8529/19/© 2019 Elsevier Inc. All rights reserved.

endo.theclinics.com

of pregnant women (752 in total) receiving antenatal care at the Boston City Hospital. The mean and standard deviation (SD) of the venous whole blood glucose concentrations for each sample, fasting and 1, 2, and 3 hours after consumption of the glucose load, were calculated. Values equal to or greater than 2 SD above the mean were considered abnormal, and it was arbitrarily decided that for the test to be called abnormal, 2 or more values should be elevated. These test criteria when applied to 1013 women followed serially for 8 years after having a 100-g OGTT during pregnancy were strongly associated with the development of diabetes during follow-up. Glucose concentrations were later extrapolated from the whole blood values measured in this study to approximate plasma glucose values for contemporary analytical methods.

In 1978, the American College of Obstetricians and Gynecologists (ACOG) recommended screening pregnant women for diabetes among individuals with historical risk factors for diabetes[2] using an OGTT interpreted by the criteria of O'Sullivan and Mahan[1] or Mestman and colleagues.[3] In 1979, the National Diabetes Data Group (NDDG)[4] published guidelines for the classification of diabetes and various categories of glucose intolerance including gestational diabetes, which was restricted to women in whom the "onset or recognition of diabetes or impaired glucose tolerance occurred during pregnancy." This subsequently became the standard definition of GDM. Interpretation of the OGTT using the criteria of O'Sullivan and Mahan[1] extrapolated for plasma values was recommended because data were unavailable to link maternal glycemia to perinatal outcomes. The World Health Organization (WHO)[5,6] also published criteria for diabetes and impaired glucose tolerance during pregnancy that were the same as values used in nonpregnant persons. Many other detection strategies and diagnostic criteria for GDM have been published.[7]

Gestational Diabetes Mellitus in the Twenty-first Century

It has been well documented and generally accepted that women found to have GDM are at high risk for development of type 2 diabetes mellitus (T2DM) in subsequent years.[1,8,9] Nevertheless, there was vigorous debate about the value of detecting and treating GDM that persisted into the twenty-first century.[10] One issue was whether the adverse perinatal outcomes in pregnancies of women with hyperglycemia less than diagnostic of diabetes mellitus are independently associated with maternal glycemia or attributable to greater obesity, higher maternal age, more urinary tract infections, or social disadvantages. The second was whether treating hyperglycemia in women with GDM actually reduced adverse outcomes.

Maternal glycemia and perinatal outcomes

The Hyperglycemia and Adverse Pregnancy Outcome (HAPO) study,[11] a multicenter, multinational, multiethnic group observational study addressed the first issue. In the HAPO study, more than 25,500 pregnant women at 15 centers in 9 countries consented to have a 75-g, 2-h OGTT at 24 to 32 weeks (mean 28) of gestation. Those with 1 or more OGTT values above or below predefined concentrations were excluded, as were those who delivered at a hospital other than where they entered the study. In the remainder, results of the OGTT were blinded to caregivers and participants, and all were given normal obstetric and neonatal care. The associations among fasting, 1-h and 2-h OGTT glucose concentrations, and 4 primary (birthweight and cord blood c-peptide each >95th percentile and rates of primary cesarean delivery and clinically recognized neonatal hypoglycemia) and several secondary outcomes were examined in 23,316 pregnancies. As illustrated in **Fig. 1**, rates of each outcome increased as each OGTT value increased. The associations were continuous and linear in models adjusted for confounders, including maternal age, body mass

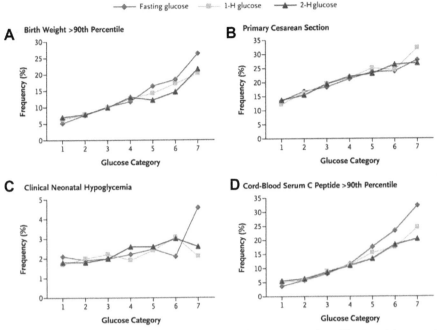

Fasting glucose — 1-H glucose — 2-H glucose

A Birth Weight >90th Percentile
B Primary Cesarean Section
C Clinical Neonatal Hypoglycemia
D Cord-Blood Serum C Peptide >90th Percentile

Fig. 1. Frequency of primary outcomes across the glucose categories of fasting, 1-hour, and 2-hour values in a 75-g OGTT. (*A*) Birth weight >90th percentile. (*B*) Primary cesarean delivery. (*C*) Clinical neonatal hypoglycemia. (*D*) Cord blood serum c-peptide >90th percentile. (*From* HAPO Study Cooperative Research Group, Metzger BE, Lowe LP, et al. Hyperglycemia and adverse pregnancy outcomes. N Engl J Med 2008;358(19):1991–2002; with permission.)

index (BMI), and study field center. There were no obvious thresholds at which risks increased. Significant associations were also observed for secondary outcomes, although these tended to be weaker.

Results of treating gestational diabetes mellitus
The impact of treating "mild" gestational diabetes has been examined in 2 randomized controlled trials (RCT). The Australian Carbohydrate Intolerance Study in Pregnant Women (ACHOIS) trial[12] reported study outcomes in 1000 women who met the then standard WHO criteria for gestational diabetes,[5,6] that is, fasting plasma glucose (FPG) <140 mg/dL and 2-h OGTT value between 140 and 199 mg/dL. The Maternal-Fetal Medicine Units Network Study[13] reported perinatal outcomes in 958 participants who met the Carpenter-Coustan criteria for gestational diabetes[14] whose FPG was less than 95 mg/dL. Although the diagnostic tests and criteria used in the 2 RCTs differed substantially, treatment outcomes were quite similar (**Table 1**), providing strong evidence that treating GDM can indeed reduce adverse pregnancy outcomes.

Diagnostic criteria, detection, and prevalence of gestational diabetes mellitus
The International Association of Diabetes and Pregnancy Study Groups (IADPSG) recommended criteria for the diagnosis of GDM that are based on the HAPO study results, supported by other evidence.[15] The IADPSG diagnostic thresholds are the first criteria based on risks of adverse perinatal outcomes, rather than risk of subsequent development of maternal diabetes[1] or by applying thresholds that define impaired glucose tolerance outside of pregnancy.[5,6]

Table 1
Treatment of mild gestational diabetes mellitus reduces adverse outcomes

Outcome	ACHOIS[a]	MFMU[b]
Birth weight	↓	↓
Large for gestational age	↓	↓
Macrosomia	↓	↓
Preeclampsia	↓	↓
Cesarean delivery	—	↓
Shoulder dystocia	—	↓

—, indicates no difference between outcome in the intervention and observation participants.
↓, indicates reduced outcome rate or mean.
[a] Australian Carbohydrate Intolerance Study.[12]
[b] Maternal Fetal Medicine Unit Network Study.[13]
Data from Crowther CA, Hiller JE, Moss JR, et al. Effect of treatment of gestational diabetes mellitus on pregnancy outcomes. N Engl J Med. 2005;352(24):2477-2486 and Landon MB, Spong CY, Thom E, et al. A multicenter, randomized trial of treatment for mild gestational diabetes. N Engl J Med. 2009;361(14):1339-1348

The 1-step approach to detection and diagnosis of GDM recommended by the IADPSG[15] results in a higher prevalence of GDM than other strategies, particularly the 2-step approaches based on the original O'Sullivan-Mahan criteria.[1] The fact that the IADPSG criteria for GDM require 1 or more rather than 2 or more OGTT values equal to or greater than defined threshold concentrations is a major reason for the higher prevalence rates. When the IADPSG criteria were applied to the HAPO study cohort retrospectively, 17.8% had GDM, and there was substantial center-to-center variation in prevalence.[16] Given the high rates of combined T2DM and prediabetes and obesity in nonpregnant women of reproductive age (**Table 2**),

Table 2
Weighted distribution and glucose and BMI categories among women age 20–44 years, United States, 1976–1980 and 2007–2010

	Weighted Percent (Standard Error)	
Diabetes/BMI status[a]	1976–1980	2007–2010
Diagnosed diabetes[b]	1.2 (0.20)	2.3 (0.29)
Undiagnosed diabetes[c]	1.2 (0.40)	2.6 (0.48)
Undiagnosed prediabetes[c]	11.9 (1.15)	24.0 (1.87)
Normal glucose levels[c]	85.8 (1.23)	71.2 (2.11)
Obese	12.1 (1.05)	32.7 (1.79)
Overweight	21.6 (1.67)	26.4 (1.67)
Normal	66.3 (1.80)	40.9 (2.30)

Women currently pregnant were excluded from the analysis.
Abbreviation: BMI, body mass index (weight/height in kg/m^2).
[a] BMI is defined as obese ($\geq$30 kg/m^2). Overweight (25 to <30 kg/m^2), normal (<25 kg/m^2).
[b] Diagnosed diabetes is self-reported.
[c] Undiagnosed diabetes, prediabetes, and normal glucose levels are defined by fasting plasma glucose or 2-hour plasma glucose from an oral glucose tolerance test using American Diabetes Association cutpoints.
From Metzger BE, Buchanan TA. Gestational diabetes. In: Cowie CC, CS, Menke A, Cissell MA, Eberhardt MS, Meigs JB, Gregg EW, Knowler WC, Barrett-Connor E, Becker DJ, Brancati FL, Boyko EJ, Herman WH, Howard BV, Narayan KMV, Rewers M, Fradkin JE, ed. Diabetes in America, 3rd ed. Bethesda, MD: National Institutes of Health, NIH Pub No. 17-1468; 2018:4-1-17.

it is not unexpected that rates of GDM are now much higher than when GDM was first recognized.[1]

Current Recommendations

The WHO has adopted the IADPSG criteria for GDM.[17] However, an independent panel of health professionals and public representatives appointed by the National Institutes of Health did not.[18] ACOG continues to recommend the traditional approach to detection and diagnosis of GDM. The high prevalence of GDM with associated costs of providing treatment and the lack of RCT data indicating benefit of treating individuals who meet IADPSG but not Carpenter-Coustan criteria for GDM (one or more values equal to or greater than the diagnostic threshold rather than two) contributed to the panel's conclusions. Thus, multiple criteria for the diagnosis of GDM are now accepted for use in the United States (**Table 3**). It remains to be seen what impact reports of benefit from treating GDM meeting IADPSG but not Carpenter-Coustan criteria for GDM[19] have on clinical practice.

OFFSPRING OUTCOMES

Perinatal and long-term offspring outcomes following exposure to diabetes in pregnancy are directly related to glycemic control during pregnancy.[11,20–22] Despite recent improvements in maternal glycemic control and a reduction in the frequency of perinatal complications, the prevalence of adverse pregnancy outcomes continues to be higher than the general population.[12,23]

Adverse Outcomes by Age Group

Potential adverse offspring outcomes vary by age group (**Table 4**) and avoidance of one outcome does not indicate reduction in risk of other adverse outcomes.[21,24,25] It is necessary to emphasize that most studies reporting short-term and long-term offspring outcomes were composed of mothers with some or all types of diabetes in pregnancy.

Table 3
Diagnosis of gestational diabetes

Glucose Value, mg/dL	100 g Oral Glucose Load[a]		Carpenter-Coustan[14] Plasma-Glucose Oxidase[d]	75 g Oral Glucose Load IADPSG[15] Plasma Enzymatic[e]
	O'Sullivan-Mahan[1] Whole Blood[b]	NDDG[4] Plasma-Autoanalyzer[c]		
Fasting	90	105	95	92
1-h	165	190	180	180
2-h	145	165	155	153
3-h	125	145	140	NA

Abbreviations: IADPSG, International Association of Diabetes and Pregnancy Study Groups; NDDG, National Diabetes Data Group.
[a] The oral glucose tolerance test should be performed in the morning after an overnight fast of at least 8 hours but not more than 14 hours and after at least 3 days of unrestricted diet ($\geq$150 g carbohydrate per day) and physical activity.
[b] For the diagnosis, 2 or more of the glucose values must be met or exceeded.[1]
[c] For the diagnosis, 2 or more of the glucose values must be met or exceeded.[4]
[d] For the diagnosis, 2 or more of the glucose values must be met or exceeded.[14]
[e] For the diagnosis, 1 or more of the glucose values must be met or exceeded.[15]

Table 4
Potential adverse outcomes in offspring exposed to gestational diabetes mellitus

Fetus	Malformations, stillbirth, chorioamnionitis, birth asphyxia, preterm birth, macrosomia
Neonate	Large for gestational age, birth injury, hypoglycemia, respiratory distress syndrome/transient tachypnea, polycythemia and hyperbilirubinemia, hypocalcemia
Child	Neurodevelopmental impairments, obesity, increased adiposity, insulin resistance, impaired glucose tolerance
Adult	Obesity, insulin resistance, impaired glucose tolerance, type 2 diabetes mellitus

Neonatal Complications

Birth complications, including high risk of cesarean delivery, shoulder dystocia, and birth injury, are often due to a large-size fetus. The Pedersen hypothesis,[26] which was later expanded on by Freinkel,[27] proposed that increased fetal size is the direct result of excessive circulating maternal glucose and other fuels that cross the placenta to provide the fetus with energy substrates. The fetus responds to excessive energy substrates by producing higher amounts of insulin, that is, fetal hyperinsulinemia, which then leads to a number of consequences, notably excessive fetal growth and subsequent large for gestational age birth size. In pregnancies complicated by diabetes, fetal insulin binds to the insulinlike growth factor 1 receptor with affinity equal to the insulin receptor.[28] Growth factors, not growth hormone, are key promoters of fetal growth.

A relative fetal hypoxia occurs in utero, which may underlie the risk of stillbirth and birth asphyxia.[29] This hypoxia induces increased erythropoietin production and subsequent polycythemia and hyperbilirubinemia in the neonate.[30] Fetal hyperinsulinemia alters lung surfactant synthesis, and this predisposes to respiratory distress syndrome,[31] a life-threatening condition in the neonatal period that leads to significant morbidity and admission to the neonatal intensive care unit.

Hypoglycemia of the neonate is a well-recognized complication in offspring of women with GDM.[32] When the constant maternal flow of glucose is abruptly halted at delivery, the relative fetal hyperinsulinemia continues and uses available neonatal glucose stores, which can lead to neonatal hypoglycemia. Preventive strategies to diagnose and treat neonatal hypoglycemia include blood glucose monitoring protocols and frequent feedings in those neonates deemed at increased risk. In the majority of instances, the condition is self-limited as the hyperinsulinemia resolves.

Large size at birth is common in offspring born to women with GDM. Numerous studies in this population have demonstrated that the increased birth weight is due to higher amounts of fat mass as opposed to fat-free muscle mass.[33,34]

Childhood Complications

Only recently has the finding of excessive adiposity among GDM offspring been documented in childhood.[21] Other long-term complications are insulin resistance, impaired glucose tolerance, and T2DM, collectively termed disorders of glucose metabolism, and psychological and developmental effects that may be related to neonatal hypoglycemia.

Risk of impaired neurodevelopmental outcomes among offspring of mothers with GDM has been studied in several cohorts.[35] Expressive language, memory recall, and facial recognition are developmental areas studied in which offspring of mothers with GDM differ from controls not exposed to GDM.[36,37] An increased risk of autism spectrum disorders in offspring of mothers with GDM also has been documented.[38]

The 2 well-described long-term follow-up studies of diabetes in pregnancy, in the Pima Indian population and at Northwestern University, documented higher rates of obesity, as measured by weight alone, among children exposed to diabetes in pregnancy compared with children not exposed.[22,39] Large birth weight was not a universal finding among these offspring.[40] Interestingly, the timing of obesity development was different in these 2 cohorts: among Pima Indians, offspring of diabetic mothers weighed more compared with offspring of nondiabetic mothers at every age throughout childhood,[40] whereas in the Northwestern cohort, obesity among offspring of mothers with diabetes emerged in the peri-pubertal years.[41] Studies among sibling pairs in the Pima Indian population born before versus after the maternal diagnosis of diabetes provide convincing evidence that the diabetic intrauterine environment underlies the elevated obesity risk, separate or perhaps additive to the genetic risk.[42] This finding of increased obesity rates among the younger siblings born after the maternal development of diabetes was duplicated in a study of Swedish male siblings.[43]

Disentangling the independent effects of maternal hyperglycemia and obesity on offspring obesity risk is important to guide preventive strategies. The HAPO Follow-up Study (FUS) demonstrated that offspring exposed to mild, untreated maternal hyperglycemia had higher rates of adiposity at a mean age of 11.4 years.[21] These results were somewhat attenuated by maternal BMI. This study, along with others,[44,45] extended earlier findings of higher weight among offspring of mothers with diabetes by demonstrating specific increases in adipose tissue using several methodologies, including skinfold thicknesses with calipers, waist circumference, dual-energy X-ray absorptiometry, and air displacement plethysmography. Higher adiposity, as opposed to higher weight, is an important risk factor for cardiometabolic diseases and early death.

HAPO is unique compared with other studies of hyperglycemia in pregnancy in that the data are not confounded by maternal treatment. Another novel finding of the HAPO FUS was that maternal hyperglycemia during pregnancy was independently associated with risk of abnormal glucose tolerance in the offspring.[46] In addition, disposition index, a predictor of T2DM, was significantly lower among offspring of mothers with GDM.[47] Several studies of T2DM in youth found high rates of exposure to maternal GDM.[47,48] However, the a priori associations in HAPO FUS between maternal GDM and offspring disorders of glucose metabolism provide further convincing evidence that in utero exposure to hyperglycemia adversely programs the fetal pancreas and increases future risk of disorders of glucose metabolism.

Summary

With the increasing prevalence of obesity among women of reproductive age, rates of GDM will continue to increase. Most concerning is the perpetuation of the cycle of diabetes between mother and child. Increased rates of adiposity and disorders of glucose metabolism in peripubertal offspring of mothers with mild, untreated GDM have been demonstrated.[21] In studies of young children whose mothers had mild GDM, there was no difference in obesity rates in the offspring of treated mothers compared with untreated mothers.[49] However, it remains to be determined whether increased obesity rates will emerge in the untreated offspring in later childhood or adolescence.

In summary, optimizing diagnosis and treatment of GDM is a necessary strategy to prevent adverse metabolic health outcomes in offspring.

TREATMENT
Lifestyle Interventions

Medical nutrition therapy (MNT) is a cornerstone of therapy for all women with GDM, and approximately 80% to 90% of women are able to meet therapeutic targets with MNT alone.[12,13] Multiple benefits have been attributed to lifestyle interventions, including decreased risk of macrosomia, decreased neonatal adiposity, and increased likelihood to achieve postpartum weight goals.[12,13,50] Generally women are advised to eat 3 small to moderate-sized meals and 2 to 3 snacks that are balanced in whole-grain carbohydrates, protein, and unsaturated fats. Because carbohydrate intolerance can be more marked at the morning meal, women are often advised to eat less carbohydrate at breakfast (for example, 30 g at breakfast compared with 45–60 g at lunch and dinner). Although evidence supporting a particular macronutrient distribution is sparse,[51] benefits of a low-glycemic index diet have been demonstrated.[52,53] Meal planning focuses not only on prescribed carbohydrate amounts and distribution, but also on pairing intake of carbohydrate with ingestion of lean protein and/or unsaturated fat at meals and snacks, to lessen the degree of postprandial carbohydrate-induced glycemic excursion. Women are frequently advised to consume a bedtime snack to counteract the greater tendency toward accelerated starvation and accompanying ketosis that characterizes the pregnant state and can emerge during the overnight fast. Stemming from literature suggesting adverse neurodevelopmental impact of gestational ketonemia,[35] some centers advise women to monitor urine ketone levels to assess for deficiency in carbohydrate intake; when ketonuria occurs, women are advised to augment nutritional intake.

Moderate physical activity is also recommended as part of the treatment program. Generally, women with GDM are advised to obtain 30 minutes of moderate-intensity aerobic exercise on at least 5 days per week or a minimum of 150 minutes over the course of the week,[54] similar to recommendations for nonpregnant people with DM. Although studies evaluating glycemic impact of exercise in GDM are sparse, exercise has been shown to improve fasting and postprandial glycemia in GDM.[55] Acute bouts of moderate-intensity walking after eating improved postprandial glucose control for up to 3 hours after the meal,[56] and post-meal walking is frequently recommended when there are no contraindications to physical activity.[54]

Pharmacologic Therapy

Insulin

When glycemic goals are not met with MNT, pharmacologic therapy is added. Insulin therapy is considered the first-line pharmacologic therapy for GDM, as it does not cross the placenta to a significant degree.[54,57] Fasting hyperglycemia is treated with basal (long-acting or intermediate-acting) insulin, and postprandial hyperglycemia is treated with prandial (rapid-acting) insulin. Basal and prandial insulin may be used separately or in combination, depending on the individual glycemic profile. General total daily insulin requirements by gestational age are shown in **Table 5**, but in practice, individual insulin requirements vary significantly, with some women achieving glycemic targets at significantly lower doses and others requiring significantly more. Weekly (or more frequent) insulin dose adjustments are made based on self-monitored glycemic patterns.

Table 5
Calculating total daily insulin requirement of a pregnant woman during different trimesters of pregnancy

Weeks Gestation	Total Daily Insulin Requirement (units/day)
1–13	Pregnant woman's weight in kg $\times$ 0.7
14–26	Pregnant woman's weight in kg $\times$ 0.8
27–37	Pregnant woman's weight in kg $\times$ 0.9
38 to delivery	Pregnant woman's weight in kg $\times$ 1.0

Based on average total daily insulin requirements in pregnant women with preexisting diabetes mellitus.

From Castorino K, Paband R, Zisser H, et al. Insulin pumps in pregnancy: using technology to achieve normoglycemia in women with diabetes. Curr Diab Rep. 2012;12(1):53-59; with permission.

NPH has long been considered the mainstay of basal insulin treatment during pregnancy due to its long track record of safety and effectiveness, but more recently, basal insulin analogs have gained increasing acceptance. Insulin detemir was shown to be noninferior to NPH in pregnancies complicated by type 1 diabetes mellitus (T1DM).[58] In addition, the rapid-acting insulin analogs aspart and lispro have acceptable safety and efficacy profiles in pregnancy.[59,60] Rapid-acting insulin analogs are generally preferred over regular insulin for prandial coverage because of their more rapid onset of action, enabling administration in closer proximity to the meal and improved postprandial glycemia.

Oral agents
At the current time, treatment of GDM with oral agents is controversial, and data on long-term outcomes for the offspring are lacking.

Glyburide Although glyburide was previously thought not to cross the placenta in significant amounts,[61] more recent studies using more sensitive assays have demonstrated significant and highly variable transplacental transfer of glyburide.[62,63] Although similar glycemic control has been reported with glyburide compared with insulin use,[61] recent data have raised concern about increased risk of adverse outcomes with use of glyburide compared with insulin, including increased risk of macrosomia[64] and neonatal hypoglycemia.[64,65] A recent RCT failed to show noninferiority of glyburide compared with insulin in the reduction of perinatal complications.[66] Long-term safety data among offspring prenatally exposed to glyburide are lacking.

Metformin Metformin freely crosses the placenta, and the fetal metformin concentration is similar to or higher than the maternal concentration.[67,68] Metformin compared with insulin use has been associated with mixed outcomes; for example, less maternal weight gain, lower postprandial glucose, and less pregnancy-induced hypertension, but higher rates of preterm birth.[64] Although short-term studies of neurodevelopmental outcomes among metformin-exposed offspring have been reassuring,[69] the potential long-term effects on fetal developmental metabolic programming and the long-term metabolic consequences in the offspring are currently unknown.[70] Notably, 2 studies reported that metformin-exposed children of mothers with polycystic ovary syndrome or GDM were found to weigh more at 4[71] and 9 years of age.[72] It is also worth noting the significant treatment failure rate observed with metformin use: up to one-half of women treated with metformin still required adjunctive insulin therapy.[64,73]

Summary

At the current time, the comparative advantages and disadvantages of insulin, glyburide, and metformin in the treatment of GDM are uncertain, especially with regard to long-term outcomes in prenatally exposed offspring. Embodying these uncertainties, current expert guidelines provide contradictory recommendations. ACOG[54] and the American Diabetes Association (ADA)[57] both recommend insulin as the preferred first-line pharmacologic therapy for GDM, whereas the Society for Maternal Fetal Medicine advises that metformin is a reasonable and safe first-line pharmacologic alternative to insulin.[74] ACOG[54] notes that oral agents (with metformin preferred over glyburide) are a reasonable alternative for women unable or unwilling to use insulin.

In our opinion, at the current time, insulin remains the first-line treatment for GDM due to the known transplacental passage of oral agents, the absence of long-term safety data in prenatally exposed offspring, and concerns about nonequivalent perinatal outcomes. This position is consistent with the ADA's current clinical practice recommendations.[57] Women should be informed that oral agents cross the placenta and that, although no prohibitive adverse fetal outcomes have been observed in short-term studies, long-term safety data are lacking.

Glucose Monitoring

Women are asked to monitor capillary blood glucose fasting and either 1 or 2 hours after meals (with selective use of pre-lunch and pre-dinner values) to guide insulin dose adjustments.

Although continuous glucose monitoring (CGM) has been shown to improve glycemic and neonatal outcomes in pregnancies complicated by T1DM,[75] studies evaluating CGM use in GDM are limited. Although improved glycemic control and pregnancy outcomes have been reported with CGM use among women with GDM,[76] these findings have not been consistent.[77] Larger studies evaluating the role of CGM use in pregnancies complicated by GDM are needed.

Glycemic Goals

The second and third trimesters of pregnancy are characterized by a progressive increase in insulin resistance and therefore insulin requirements because of the gradual increase in placental elaboration of diabetogenic hormones over the course of gestation. As a result, frequent glucose monitoring and therapeutic adjustments are typically required to achieve glycemic targets.

Glycemic targets are as follows[54,57]:

- Fasting less than 95 mg/dL (5.3 mmol/L) and either
- One-hour postprandial less than 140 mg/dL (7.8 mmol/L) or
- Two-hour postprandial less than 120 mg/dL (6.7 mmol/L)

Women are advised to submit weekly glucose updates. Typically, changes to the therapeutic regimen (addition of insulin for those treated with lifestyle modifications only, or adjustment of the insulin regimen for those already taking insulin) are recommended when 20% to 25% of glucose values (e.g., 2 days out of 7) at a particular time point (fasting and/or following a particular meal) are above target despite adherence to the existing treatment regimen, or if hypoglycemia occurs. Serial adjustments to the basal and/or prandial insulin doses are guided by patterns in self-monitored glucose levels, individually or in combination. In addition to insulin doses, ongoing attention is paid to the impact on glycemic patterns of other factors, including timing of prandial insulin administration in relation to food intake,[78] meal composition/food choices, and physical activity.

REFERENCES

1. O'Sullivan JB, Mahan CM. Criteria for the oral glucose tolerance test in pregnancy. Diabetes 1964;13:278–85.
2. American College of Obstetricians and Gynecologists. Management of diabetes mellitus in pregnancy. Technical Bulletin no. 48. Washington, DC: ACOG; 1978.
3. Mestman JH, Anderson GV, Barton P. Carbohydrate metabolism in pregnancy. A study of 658 patients with the use of the oral glucose tolerance test and the prednisolone glucose tolerance test. Am J Obstet Gynecol 1971;109(1):41–5.
4. Classification and diagnosis of diabetes mellitus and other categories of glucose intolerance. National Diabetes Data Group. Diabetes 1979;28(12):1039–57.
5. WHO Expert Committee on Diabetes Mellitus: second report. World Health Organ Tech Rep Ser 1980;646:1–80.
6. Diabetes mellitus. Report of a WHO Study Group. World Health Organ Tech Rep Ser 1985;727:1–113.
7. Cutchie WA, Cheung NW, Simmons D. Comparison of international and New Zealand guidelines for the care of pregnant women with diabetes. Diabet Med 2006; 23(5):460–8.
8. Kim C, Newton KM, Knopp RH. Gestational diabetes and the incidence of type 2 diabetes: a systematic review. Diabetes Care 2002;25(10):1862–8.
9. Metzger BE. Long-term outcomes in mothers diagnosed with gestational diabetes mellitus and their offspring. Clin Obstet Gynecol 2007;50(4):972–9.
10. Metzger BE, Buchanan TA. Gestational diabetes. In: Cowie CC, Casagrande SS, Menke A, et al, editors. Diabetes in America. 3rd edition. Bethesda (MD): National Institutes of Health; 2018. p. 1–17.
11. Metzger BE, Lowe LP, Dyer AR, et al. Hyperglycemia and adverse pregnancy outcomes. N Engl J Med 2008;358(19):1991–2002.
12. Crowther CA, Hiller JE, Moss JR, et al. Effect of treatment of gestational diabetes mellitus on pregnancy outcomes. N Engl J Med 2005;352(24):2477–86.
13. Landon MB, Spong CY, Thom E, et al. A multicenter, randomized trial of treatment for mild gestational diabetes. N Engl J Med 2009;361(14):1339–48.
14. Carpenter MW, Coustan DR. Criteria for screening tests for gestational diabetes. Am J Obstet Gynecol 1982;144(7):768–73.
15. International Association of Diabetes Pregnancy Study Groups Consensus Panel, Metzger BE, Gabbe SG, Persson B, et al. International Association of Diabetes and pregnancy study groups recommendations on the diagnosis and classification of hyperglycemia in pregnancy. Diabetes Care 2010;33(3):676–82.
16. Sacks DA, Hadden DR, Maresh M, et al. Frequency of gestational diabetes mellitus at collaborating centers based on IADPSG consensus panel-recommended criteria: the Hyperglycemia and Adverse Pregnancy Outcome (HAPO) Study. Diabetes Care 2012;35(3):526–8.
17. Diagnostic criteria and classification of hyperglycaemia first detected in pregnancy: a World Health Organization guideline. Diabetes Res Clin Pract 2014; 103(3):341–63.
18. National Institutes of Health consensus development conference statement: diagnosing gestational diabetes mellitus, March 4-6, 2013. Obstet Gynecol 2013; 122(2 Pt 1):358–69.

19. Yang X, Tian H, Zhang F, et al. A randomised translational trial of lifestyle intervention using a 3-tier shared care approach on pregnancy outcomes in Chinese women with gestational diabetes mellitus but without diabetes. J Transl Med 2014;12:290.

20. Falavigna M, Schmidt MI, Trujillo J, et al. Effectiveness of gestational diabetes treatment: a systematic review with quality of evidence assessment. Diabetes Res Clin Pract 2012;98(3):396–405.

21. Lowe WL Jr, Scholtens DM, Lowe LP, et al. Association of gestational diabetes with maternal disorders of glucose metabolism and childhood adiposity. JAMA 2018;320(10):1005–16.

22. Pettitt DJ, Knowler WC. Long-term effects of the intrauterine environment, birth weight, and breast-feeding in Pima Indians. Diabetes Care 1998;21(Suppl 2): B138–41.

23. Wexler DJ, Powe CE, Barbour LA, et al. Research gaps in gestational diabetes mellitus: executive summary of a National Institute of Diabetes and Digestive and Kidney Diseases workshop. Obstet Gynecol 2018;132(2):496–505.

24. Schaefer-Graf UM, Buchanan TA, Xiang A, et al. Patterns of congenital anomalies and relationship to initial maternal fasting glucose levels in pregnancies complicated by type 2 and gestational diabetes. Am J Obstet Gynecol 2000;182(2): 313–20.

25. Wendland EM, Torloni MR, Falavigna M, et al. Gestational diabetes and pregnancy outcomes—a systematic review of the World Health Organization (WHO) and the International Association of Diabetes in Pregnancy Study Groups (IADPSG) diagnostic criteria. BMC Pregnancy Childbirth 2012;12:23.

26. Pedersen J. Weight and length at birth of infants of diabetic mothers. Acta Endocrinol (Copenh) 1954;16(4):330–42.

27. Freinkel N. Banting lecture 1980. of pregnancy and progeny. Diabetes 1980; 29(12):1023–35.

28. Hiden U, Glitzner E, Hartmann M, et al. Insulin and the IGF system in the human placenta of normal and diabetic pregnancies. J Anat 2009;215(1):60–8.

29. Dudley DJ. Diabetic-associated stillbirth: incidence, pathophysiology, and prevention. Obstet Gynecol Clin North Am 2007;34(2):293–307, ix.

30. Salvesen DR, Brudenell JM, Snijders RJ, et al. Fetal plasma erythropoietin in pregnancies complicated by maternal diabetes mellitus. Am J Obstet Gynecol 1993;168(1 Pt 1):88–94.

31. Moore TR. A comparison of amniotic fluid fetal pulmonary phospholipids in normal and diabetic pregnancy. Am J Obstet Gynecol 2002;186(4):641–50.

32. Metzger BE, Persson B, Lowe LP, et al. Hyperglycemia and adverse pregnancy outcome study: neonatal glycemia. Pediatrics 2010;126(6):e1545–52.

33. Sewell MF, Huston-Presley L, Super DM, et al. Increased neonatal fat mass, not lean body mass, is associated with maternal obesity. Am J Obstet Gynecol 2006;195(4):1100–3.

34. HAPO Study Cooperative Research Group. Hyperglycemia and Adverse Pregnancy Outcome (HAPO) Study: associations with neonatal anthropometrics. Diabetes 2009;58(2):453–9.

35. Rizzo TA, Dooley SL, Metzger BE, et al. Prenatal and perinatal influences on long-term psychomotor development in offspring of diabetic mothers. Am J Obstet Gynecol 1995;173(6):1753–8.

36. Fraser A, Nelson SM, Macdonald-Wallis C, et al. Associations of existing diabetes, gestational diabetes, and glycosuria with offspring IQ and educational

attainment: the Avon Longitudinal Study of Parents and Children. Exp Diabetes Res 2012;2012:963735.

37. Dionne G, Boivin M, Seguin JR, et al. Gestational diabetes hinders language development in offspring. Pediatrics 2008;122(5):e1073–9.

38. Nahum Sacks K, Friger M, Shoham-Vardi I, et al. Prenatal exposure to gestational diabetes mellitus as an independent risk factor for long-term neuropsychiatric morbidity of the offspring. Am J Obstet Gynecol 2016;215(3):380.e1-7.

39. Silverman BL, Rizzo TA, Cho NH, et al. Long-term effects of the intrauterine environment. The Northwestern University Diabetes in Pregnancy Center. Diabetes Care 1998;21(Suppl 2):B142–9.

40. Pettitt DJ, Knowler WC, Bennett PH, et al. Obesity in offspring of diabetic Pima Indian women despite normal birth weight. Diabetes Care 1987;10(1):76–80.

41. Silverman BL, Rizzo T, Green OC, et al. Long-term prospective evaluation of offspring of diabetic mothers. Diabetes 1991;40(Suppl 2):121–5.

42. Dabelea D, Hanson RL, Lindsay RS, et al. Intrauterine exposure to diabetes conveys risks for type 2 diabetes and obesity: a study of discordant sibships. Diabetes 2000;49(12):2208–11.

43. Lawlor DA, Lichtenstein P, Langstrom N. Association of maternal diabetes mellitus in pregnancy with offspring adiposity into early adulthood: sibling study in a prospective cohort of 280,866 men from 248,293 families. Circulation 2011; 123(3):258–65.

44. Zhao P, Liu E, Qiao Y, et al. Maternal gestational diabetes and childhood obesity at age 9-11: results of a multinational study. Diabetologia 2016;59(11):2339–48.

45. Vohr BR, McGarvey ST, Tucker R. Effects of maternal gestational diabetes on offspring adiposity at 4-7 years of age. Diabetes Care 1999;22(8):1284–91.

46. Tam WH, Ma RCW, Ozaki R, et al. In utero exposure to maternal hyperglycemia increases childhood cardiometabolic risk in offspring. Diabetes Care 2017; 40(5):679–86.

47. Holder T, Giannini C, Santoro N, et al. A low disposition index in adolescent offspring of mothers with gestational diabetes: a risk marker for the development of impaired glucose tolerance in youth. Diabetologia 2014;57(11):2413–20.

48. Dabelea D, Mayer-Davis EJ, Lamichhane AP, et al. Association of intrauterine exposure to maternal diabetes and obesity with type 2 diabetes in youth: the SEARCH Case-Control Study. Diabetes Care 2008;31(7):1422–6.

49. Landon MB, Rice MM, Varner MW, et al. Mild gestational diabetes mellitus and long-term child health. Diabetes Care 2015;38(3):445–52.

50. Brown J, Alwan NA, West J, et al. Lifestyle interventions for the treatment of women with gestational diabetes. Cochrane Database Syst Rev 2017;(5):CD011970.

51. Han S, Middleton P, Shepherd E, et al. Different types of dietary advice for women with gestational diabetes mellitus. Cochrane Database Syst Rev 2017;(2):CD009275.

52. Viana LV, Gross JL, Azevedo MJ. Dietary intervention in patients with gestational diabetes mellitus: a systematic review and meta-analysis of randomized clinical trials on maternal and newborn outcomes. Diabetes Care 2014;37(12):3345–55.

53. Wei J, Heng W, Gao J. Effects of low glycemic index diets on gestational diabetes mellitus: a meta-analysis of randomized controlled clinical trials. Medicine (Baltimore) 2016;95(22):e3792.

54. Committee on Practice Bulletins-Obstetrics. ACOG Practice Bulletin No. 190: gestational diabetes mellitus. Obstet Gynecol 2018;131(2):e49–64.

55. Harrison AL, Shields N, Taylor NF, et al. Exercise improves glycaemic control in women diagnosed with gestational diabetes mellitus: a systematic review. J Physiother 2016;62(4):188–96.

56. Coe DP, Conger SA, Kendrick JM, et al. Postprandial walking reduces glucose levels in women with gestational diabetes mellitus. Appl Physiol Nutr Metab 2018;43(5):531–4.

57. American Diabetes Association. Standards of medical care in diabetes - 2019. Diabetes Care 2019;42(Supplement 1):S1–193.

58. Mathiesen ER, Hod M, Ivanisevic M, et al. Maternal efficacy and safety outcomes in a randomized, controlled trial comparing insulin detemir with NPH insulin in 310 pregnant women with type 1 diabetes. Diabetes Care 2012;35(10):2012–7.

59. Lv S, Wang J, Xu Y. Safety of insulin analogs during pregnancy: a meta-analysis. Arch Gynecol Obstet 2015;292(4):749–56.

60. Durnwald CP, Landon MB. A comparison of lispro and regular insulin for the management of type 1 and type 2 diabetes in pregnancy. J Matern Fetal Neonatal Med 2008;21(5):309–13.

61. Langer O, Conway DL, Berkus MD, et al. A comparison of glyburide and insulin in women with gestational diabetes mellitus. N Engl J Med 2000;343(16):1134–8.

62. Schwartz RA, Rosenn B, Aleksa K, et al. Glyburide transport across the human placenta. Obstet Gynecol 2015;125(3):583–8.

63. Caritis SN, Hebert MF. A pharmacologic approach to the use of glyburide in pregnancy. Obstet Gynecol 2013;121(6):1309–12.

64. Balsells M, Garcia-Patterson A, Sola I, et al. Glibenclamide, metformin, and insulin for the treatment of gestational diabetes a systematic review and meta-analysis. BMJ 2015;350:h102.

65. Song R, Chen L, Chen Y, et al. Comparison of glyburide and insulin in the management of gestational diabetes: a meta-analysis. PLoS One 2017;12(8): e0182488.

66. Senat MV, Affres H, Letourneau A, et al. Effect of glyburide vs subcutaneous insulin on perinatal complications among women with gestational diabetes: a randomized clinical trial. JAMA 2018;319(17):1773–80.

67. Eyal S, Easterling TR, Carr D, et al. Pharmacokinetics of metformin during pregnancy. Drug Metab Dispos 2010;38(5):833–40.

68. Vanky E, Zahlsen K, Spigset O, et al. Placental passage of metformin in women with polycystic ovary syndrome. Fertil Steril 2005;83(5):1575–8.

69. Wouldes TA, Battin M, Coat S, et al. Neurodevelopmental outcome at 2 years in offspring of women randomised to metformin or insulin treatment for gestational diabetes. Arch Dis Child Fetal Neonatal Ed 2016;101(6):F488–93.

70. Barbour LA, Scifres C, Valent AM, et al. A cautionary response to SMFM statement: pharmacological treatment of gestational diabetes. Am J Obstet Gynecol 2018;219(4):367.e1–e7.

71. Hanem LGE, Stridsklev S, Juliusson PB, et al. Metformin use in PCOS pregnancies increases the risk of offspring overweight at 4 years of age: follow-up of two RCTs. J Clin Endocrinol Metab 2018;103(4):1612–21.

72. Rowan JA, Rush EC, Plank LD, et al. Metformin in gestational diabetes: the offspring follow-up (MiG TOFU): body composition and metabolic outcomes at 7-9 years of age. BMJ Open Diabetes Res Care 2018;6(1):e000456.

73. Rowan JA, Hague WM, Gao W, et al. Metformin versus insulin for the treatment of gestational diabetes. N Engl J Med 2008;358(19):2003–15.

74. Society of Maternal-Fetal Medicine Publications Committee. SMFM statement: pharmacological treatment of gestational diabetes. Am J Obstet Gynecol 2018; 218(5):B2–4.

75. Feig DS, Donovan LE, Corcoy R, et al. Continuous glucose monitoring in pregnant women with type 1 diabetes (CONCEPTT): a multicentre international randomised controlled trial. Lancet 2017;390(10110):2347–59.

76. Yu F, Lv L, Liang Z, et al. Continuous glucose monitoring effects on maternal glycemic control and pregnancy outcomes in patients with gestational diabetes mellitus: a prospective cohort study. J Clin Endocrinol Metab 2014;99(12):4674–82.

77. Wei Q, Sun Z, Yang Y, et al. Effect of a CGMS and SMBG on maternal and neonatal outcomes in gestational diabetes mellitus: a randomized controlled trial. Sci Rep 2016;6:19920.

78. Murphy HR, Elleri D, Allen JM, et al. Pathophysiology of postprandial hyperglycaemia in women with type 1 diabetes during pregnancy. Diabetologia 2012; 55(2):282–93.

Type 1 Diabetes in Pregnancy

David R. McCance, MD*, Claire Casey, PhD

KEYWORDS

- Type 1 diabetes • Pregnancy • Glycemic control • Maternal/fetal outcomes

KEY POINTS

- Adverse maternal/fetal outcomes in type 1 diabetic pregnancy remain severalfold higher than in the background population.
- The benefits of pregnancy planning in improving outcomes are clear, but still only a minority of women plan their pregnancy, and education must remain a key priority.
- Recent advances in insulin delivery and glucose sensing offer promise, but elucidation of their relative roles and precise indication for use is urgently needed.

EPIDEMIOLOGY

Globally, 21.3 million (16.2%) of 131.4 million live births to women aged 20 to 49 years are affected by hyperglycemia in pregnancy.[1] Approximately 6.2% of these 21.3 million cases are due to diabetes detected before pregnancy (either type 1 diabetes [T1DM] or type 2 diabetes).[1] A UK national report in England and Wales in 2015 estimated that approximately 1500 babies were born to mothers with T1DM, and that this accounted for 0.21% of all live births.[2] The prevalence of diabetes is highest in white women.[3] The incidence of T1DM in pregnancy is lower than in the nonpregnant population, partially owing to the lower fertility; however, the gap has decreased significantly over time.[4]

ADVERSE PERINATAL/MATERNAL OUTCOMES

Women with T1DM have a 2-5fold increased risk of adverse pregnancy outcomes, including congenital anomalies, stillbirth, and perinatal mortality.[5,6] A review in 2013 of 12 population-based studies published within the previous 10 years compared 14,099 women with T1DM with 4,035,373 women from the background population[5] reported:

Disclosure: The authors have no conflicts of interest to declare.
Regional Centre for Endocrinology and Diabetes, Royal Victoria Hospital, Grosvenor Road, Belfast BT12 6BA, Northern Ireland, UK
* Corresponding author.
E-mail address: david.mccance@belfasttrust.hscni.net

- Congenital malformations, 5.0% versus 2.1% (relative risk [RR] = 2.4)
- Perinatal mortality, 2.7% versus 0.72% (RR = 3.7)
- Preterm delivery, 25.2% versus 6.0% (RR = 4.2)
- Large for gestational age (LGA) infants, 54.2% versus 10.0% (RR = 4.5)

In the 2016 UK National Diabetes in Pregnancy Audit, almost 1 in 2 babies had complications related to maternal diabetes.[7]

Risk factors for mother and baby

- General risk factors: age, parity, weight, hypertension, smoking, and drug abuse
- Obstetric risk factors: previous miscarriage, multiple pregnancy, nutritional deficiency, late booking, and poor obstetric history
  - Maternal risk: miscarriage, accelerated retinopathy and nephropathy, hypoglycemia and hypoglycemic unawareness, diabetic ketoacidosis (DKA), preeclampsia, hydramnios, operative delivery, infection
  - Fetal risk: still birth, perinatal mortality, congenital anomalies, small for gestational age (SGA)/large for gestational age (LGA), preterm delivery, operative delivery, shoulder dystocia and birth injury, neonatal hypoglycemia, polycythemia, hypocalcemia, respiratory distress syndrome

---

PATHOPHYSIOLOGY

Adaptation of maternal metabolism during pregnancy involves a greater decrease in plasma glucose and amino acids, and a greater increase in free fatty acids to overnight fasting than in the nonpregnant state ("accelerated starvation") associated with hepatic insulin resistance.[8] In later pregnancy, a progressive increase in postprandial glucose and its associated insulin response, associated with decreased insulin sensitivity, parallels the growth of the fetal placental unit, and rapidly reverses after delivery. This "facilitated anabolism" brings about appropriate changes in carbohydrate, amino acid, and lipid metabolism, and ensures an adequate supply of nutrients for the developing fetus. Deficient β-cell reserve, as in T1DM, will result in the abnormal adaptation of carbohydrate, protein, and fat metabolism. In T1DM, sufficient insulin is required to compensate for increasing caloric needs, increasing adiposity, decreasing exercise, and increasing anti-insulin hormones. The insulin dose to maintain normoglycemia and prevent maternal ketosis may increase up to 3-fold in the course of pregnancy in T1DM.[9] Placental hormones have been implicated in the cause of insulin resistance in late pregnancy, although the mechanism is not completely understood and likely to be multifactorial.[9,10]

RATIONALE FOR PREGNANCY PLANNING

Recognition that congenital malformations were increased in infants of diabetic mothers was first observed over 40 years ago and quickly linked with maternal periconceptional hyperglycemia. Most abnormalities occur in the teratologically sensitive period up until the seventh gestational week. The evidence that optimal glycemic control early during the first trimester is associated with improved outcomes, reduced congenital anomalies, and perinatal mortality, is well established.[11,12]

It is important, however, for the mother to realize that these risks are reduced with any improvement in glycosylated hemoglobin (HbA1c).[13] The most common types of malformation are cardiac and neural tube defects.

COMPONENTS OF PRE-PREGNANCY SERVICE

There are 2 separate components to education about reproductive health for women with T1DM: preconception counseling and pre-pregnancy care (PPC).[14]

Preconception counseling is the education of, and the discussion with, women of reproductive age about pregnancy and contraception. It should take place at regular intervals during a woman's reproductive years and include education and discussion on the following:

- Future pregnancy plans
- The use of contraception including the assessment of risks for each method
- Increased risks of adverse outcomes associated with poor glycemic control
- The nature of PPC and how it can improve pregnancy outcomes
- Folic acid supplementation before and during pregnancy
- The risks of smoking and alcohol consumption during pregnancy
- Avoidance of statins and angiotensin-converting enzyme (ACE) inhibitors during early pregnancy

PPC is the additional care required to prepare a woman with diabetes for pregnancy. Ideally, PPC should be delivered by a multidisciplinary team who will care for her during pregnancy and should begin at least 6 months before conception. The aim of PPC is to optimize glycemic control before conception. The content of PPC is outlined in **Box 1**.

Box 1
Aims of pre-pregnancy care for women with type 1 diabetes

Contraception
1. Document use of effective contraception
2. Continue contraception until optimum HbA1c achieved

Optimize glucose control
1. Aim for HbA1c as close to normal range as possible without significant hypoglycemia
2. Advise blood glucose monitoring before and 1 h postprandial, and occasionally during the night
   - Pre-meal glucose <5.3 mmol/L
   - Post-meals (1 h) <7.8 mmol/L
3. Stop oral hypoglycemic agents and initiate insulin if suboptimal glucose control
4. Consider metformin if improved glycemia outweighs potential risks
5. Advise on management of hypoglycemia

Diet, exercise, and structured education
1. Refer to dietitian for education on regular basis, but small to moderate portions of low-glycemic index carbohydrates
2. Education about weight loss if body mass index $\geq$27 kg/m^2
3. Encourage regular exercise
4. Provide smoking and alcohol cessation advice.

Prescribe folic acid supplements
   Supplemental dose: 5 mg daily (dose may vary)

Review other medication
1. Stop ACE inhibitors, angiotensin receptor antagonists, statins, or diuretics.
2. Treat hypertension with methyldopa or labetalol

Screen for diabetic complications
1. Assess for retinopathy at initial visit (if not assessed in previous 6 mo) and then annually. If retinopathy is present, consider referral to ophthalmologist
2. If proteinuria or reduced glomerular filtration rate is present, refer to nephrologist
3. Assess cardiac status and consider referral to cardiologist

Screen for rubella immunity

> Counsel on risks of pregnancy with diabetes and obesity
> 1. To fetus: miscarriage, malformation, stillbirth, neonatal death, macrosomia
> 2. To pregnancy: eclampsia, premature delivery, caesarean delivery
> 3. Progression of diabetic complications
>
> Consider referral to obstetrician or diabetes specialist midwife
> 1. Assessment of obstetric risk
> 2. Further education and support

Despite the clear advantages of PPC in improving outcomes, not all women with T1DM attend for PPC. Such women are more likely to be younger, with no third-level education, and not married or in a relationship.[15] Awareness of the rationale for PPC in women with T1DM has increased in recent years, even among nonattenders. In one study, the most common reason for not attending was because their pregnancy was not fully planned or that conception occurred more quickly than expected (45%). Other reasons for nonattendance at PPC were fertility concerns (31%), negative relationships with health professionals (21%), complex emotional issues (17%), including fear of being disappointed and wanting a "normal pregnancy," and logistical/financial concerns (10%).[16]

COMPLICATIONS OF PREGNANCY COMPLICATED BY TYPE 1 DIABETES
Hypoglycemia

Hypoglycemia is defined as a blood glucose level less than 4.0 mmol/L, and is a major challenge to achieving near normal blood glucose levels during pregnancy. It is subclassified as mild (self-treated) or severe (requiring assistance from another party), with both occurring more frequently during pregnancy. A literature review reported that 45% of women with T1DM experienced severe hypoglycemia during pregnancy, and this was 3 to 5 times more frequent in early pregnancy compared with immediately before pregnancy.[17] Predictors of severe hypoglycemia include impaired hypoglycemia awareness, a past history of severe hypoglycemia, a long duration of diabetes, low HbA1c in early pregnancy, fluctuating glucose levels, and excessive use of supplementary insulin between meals.[17]

There are no apparent long-term consequences of maternal hypoglycemia on human offspring. The major risks are to the woman herself and include loss of consciousness, seizures, hospital admission, and death.[18]

Retinopathy

Diabetic retinopathy is a leading cause of acquired blindness in young and middle-aged adults. The precise mechanisms of diabetic retinopathy progression during pregnancy remain unclear, but include metabolic, hormonal, hemodynamic, and immune-inflammatory theories.[19,20]

Diabetic eye screening and optimizing blood glucose control, hypertension, and serum lipids before pregnancy are essential, as is regular monitoring to detect and reduce the risk of retinopathy progression during pregnancy and in the postpartum period. Retinal screening protocols[21] usually comprise surveillance in the 6 months before pregnancy, during the first and second trimester, and postpartum, with additional assessments being directed by significant disease and/or previous treatments for diabetic retinopathy.

Hypertension/Nephropathy

Hypertension complicates 1 in 10 pregnancies, and the prevalence is even higher in women with diabetes, in whom up to 40% are reported to have a blood pressure exceeding 140/90 mm Hg.[22] There are 4 hypertensive disorders that can occur during pregnancy, all of which increase the risk of adverse pregnancy outcomes:

- Chronic hypertension (present before pregnancy or up to 20 weeks)
- Gestational hypertension (development of hypertension before 20 weeks)
- Preeclampsia (prevalence increases with degree of nephropathy: 6%–10% with normal albumin excretion; 42% with microalbuminuria; 64% with nephropathy present before/in early pregnancy)
- Diabetic nephropathy (prevalence 3%–15%)

Diabetic nephropathy affects pregnancy by 2 mechanisms:
- Development of severe maternal hypertension necessitating termination of the pregnancy and thereby preterm delivery
- Impaired placental development leading to fetal growth restriction and risk of stillbirth

Close monitoring of blood pressure (target <140/90 and even 130/85 mm Hg) is indicated at each visit along with periodic measurement of urinary albumin. In general, pregnancy outcome is favorable and there is usually no deterioration in maternal renal function if serum creatinine is less than 124 μmol/L, proteinuria is less than 1 g/24 hours, and blood pressure is normal in early pregnancy, when tight antihypertensive treatment is given. By contrast, a serum creatinine greater than 176 μmol/L, severe hypertension or proteinuria (above 3 g/L), and/or preexisting cardiovascular disease are associated with a high risk for poor maternal and fetal outcome and pregnancy-induced deterioration in maternal kidney function leading to kidney failure.[22] Methyldopa, β-adrenergic drugs (eg, labetolol), and slow-release calcium channel blockers may be used during pregnancy. ACE inhibitors and angiotensin receptor blockers are contraindicated and should be substituted before or at the latest in early pregnancy.

Diabetic Ketoacidosis

Historically, prevalence rates during pregnancy of 1% to 2% have been reported, and recent evidence would suggest that these have not diminished (2.7% in 2016 UK National Diabetes in Pregnancy Audit).[7] DKA occurs in the setting of absolute or relative insulin deficiency. Insulin deficiency leads to hyperglycemia and a rise in plasma glucagon, which in turn stimulates hepatic gluconeogenesis and lipolysis with subsequent ketogenesis. The physiologic changes that occur during pregnancy can increase the risk of ketosis and subsequent acidosis.

Protocols for the rapid diagnosis of DKA in pregnant women are similar to those in nonpregnant women, although care is needed to avoid over hydration.[23] Precipitants such as infection, systemic illness, emesis, dehydration, insulin omission, and medications (eg, tocolytics and corticosteroids) need to be identified and treated.

Studies dating back over 20 years have reported fetal mortality rates of 9% to 35%, although current rates are likely to be lower. The greatest loss occurs if the diagnosis and treatment are delayed.

Mothers with T1DM must be familiar with the "sick day" rules, including instructions on how to monitor urinary or capillary ketones, and be reminded constantly of the need for supplementary insulin as guided by intensive home blood glucose monitoring. A 24-hour emergency access to diabetes team members is essential.

MANAGEMENT OF DIABETES WITHIN PREGNANCY

The model which has been recommended for the care of pregnant women with T1DM before pregnancy is a multidisciplinary team operating in a secondary- or tertiary-care setting.[21] Members of the team include an obstetrician, an endocrinologist, a diabetes specialist midwife, a diabetes specialist nurse, and a diabetes specialist dietitian.

The overall aim of joint antenatal diabetes care is to allow the mother to have an enjoyable experience of pregnancy and delivery of a normal and healthy baby. This is best achieved by attendance for PPC (see above), referral for specialist care immediately on diagnosis of pregnancy, 2-weekly multidisciplinary reviews during pregnancy, and clear postnatal plans for contraception with early referral back to her usual diabetes team.

Pregnancy Care

Pregnancy care is designed to facilitate and advise on the following (**Box 2**):

Box 2
Pregnancy care

- Rapid referral to a joint antenatal diabetes clinic
- Blood glucose targets and the rationale for excellent glycemic control
- Cessation of any potentially teratogenic medications
- Folic acid usage
- Measurement of HbA1c to assess risk of fetal abnormalities
- Detection, monitoring, and management of diabetes-related complications
- Usual pregnancy care, for example, accurate pregnancy dating and ultrasound detection of fetal abnormalities
- Determination of the most appropriate time and mode of delivery
- Management plan for blood glucose levels post-delivery

Glycemic Targets Pre-pregnancy and During Pregnancy

Ideally, discussion regarding glycemic targets should take place in the planning stage of pregnancy. Equally important is the need to counsel the pregnant woman on the risks of hypoglycemia and its management. Women are advised to test their capillary blood glucose fasting, pre-meals, 1-hour post-meals, and at bedtime during pregnancy aiming to achieve the following glycemic targets:

Capillary monitoring glucose targets:[21,24]

- Fasting <5.3 mmol/L

    AND

- 1 hour after meals: <7.8 mmol/L

    OR

- 2 hours after meals: <6.4 mmol/L

The lower target is to maintain a capillary plasma glucose level above 4 mmol/L.[21]

HbA1c levels should be measured at the booking visit as an index of periconceptual glycemic control and as a predictor of adverse outcomes including congenital malformations.[16] The UK National Institute for Health and Care Excellence (NICE) guidance and American Diabetes Association recommends a target HbA1c of 6.0% to 6.5% (42–48 mmol/mol)[21,24] or less than 7.0% (53 mmol/mol) in patients who are susceptible to hypoglycemia.[24]

Increased levels of HbA1c in the periconceptual period and first trimester increase the risk of preeclampsia, perinatal/neonatal death, and congenital malformations.[7,13,25,26] Measurement of HbA1c during the second and third trimester of pregnancy may need to be interpreted more cautiously given altered red blood cell turnover, but high levels are associated with preeclampsia, preterm delivery, LGA, and neonatal intensive care admission.[25,26] The level of risk increases with an HbA1c level above 48 mmol/L (6.5%).[13]

The 2016 UK National Diabetes in Pregnancy Audit[7] audit confirmed that only 13% to 15% of pregnant women with T1DM achieve target HbA1c (<48 mmol/mol) in early pregnancy, rising to 35% in late pregnancy. In women with suboptimal HbA1c levels (>48 mmol/mol after 24 weeks), preterm delivery, LGA, and neonatal intensive care unit (NICU) rates exceeded 50% compared with 30% in women with optimal HbA1c levels (<48 mol/mol after 24 weeks).[7]

Time Blood Glucose Levels are in Target

Continuous Glucose Monitoring Systems (CGMS) have highlighted the fluctuation of glucose levels, including nocturnally, which may not be appreciated by conventional preprandial and postprandial capillary blood glucose monitoring.[27,28] Improved sensors, together with an evolving consensus on the expression of CGMS data, has resulted in this technology gaining acceptance as a valid clinical measure of blood glucose and as endpoint in clinical trials.[29]

The evidence to date would suggest that pregnant women with T1DM using standard pumps and pens, spend only 12 h/d with near normal glucose levels (50% time in target during pregnancy). They spend 10 h/d above the NICE recommended glucose target (3.9–7.8 mmol/L; 40% of the time too high), and 2 h/d below the target (10% of the time too low).[30] By the third trimester, maternal hyperglycemia improved only slightly even with frequent antenatal clinic visits. In addition, it is not clear that sensor-augmented pumps are better than standard pumps.

Relation of HbA1c, Preprandial, and Postprandial Glucose Levels to Maternal Fetal Outcome

Although the benefits of near normal glycemic control, both before and during pregnancy, are universally recognized, the optimal means to achieve this are unknown.

A randomized controlled trial (RCT) by Manderson and colleagues[31] showed that effectively managing postprandial glucose levels was more likely to be associated with a successful pregnancy outcome than controlling fasting glucose levels. In addition, spikes of high glucose values (>11 mmol/L [198 mg/dL]) are a strong predictor for LGA/macrosomia.[32]

MANAGEMENT OF GLYCEMIA
Insulin Regimens

Most patients with diabetes before pregnancy are now using a multiple dose insulin (MDI) regimen comprising a short-acting prandial insulin and an intermediate/long-acting insulin up to 3 times daily. Data on the safety and efficacy of analog insulins have largely come from observational studies, but a large RCT of insulin aspart versus regular soluble insulin in T1DM showed similar efficacy, with a tendency to lower rates of hypoglycemia and without apparent toxicity.[33] An RCT of 310 women with T1DM randomized to insulin detemir or NPH insulin (both with mealtime insulin aspart) revealed noninferior HbA1c values.[34] Large RCT data for insulin glargine are not available, but a review of observational studies did not show any excess of adverse outcomes.

The pharmacokinetic properties of faster aspart (fast-acting insulin aspart [Fiasp]; onset of appearance in blood stream 4 minutes) and insulin degludec (half-life 25 hours) analogs have a particular conceptual appeal in pregnancy, with their potential to reduce postprandial glycemic excursions and hypoglycemia. In nonpregnant adults with T1DM, prandial Fiasp was associated with improved 1-hour postprandial glucose levels versus aspart, and significantly reduced HbA1c, whereas a 12-month RCT of degludec/aspart versus glargine/aspart was associated with significant reduction in nocturnal hypoglycemia and HbA1c compared with glargine. Fiasp is deemed safe in pregnancy and a trial to examine the safety and efficacy of degludec is currently in progress.

Continuous Subcutaneous Insulin Infusion

There is little evidence supporting the routine use of continuous subcutaneous insulin infusion (CSII) in pregnancy. A meta-analysis of 6 studies (107 CSII vs 106 MDI) showed comparable glucose control and pregnancy outcomes,[35] although these studies were in the preanalog era, lacked power to detect differences in neonatal outcomes, and were likely to be confounded by selection bias.

The UK National Diabetes in Pregnancy Audit showed no difference in glycemic control or maternal fetal health outcomes between standard pump users (30% T1DM women) and pens (70% T1DM women), with suboptimal glucose control in both (mean HbA1c 51 vs 52 mmol/mol in pump vs pen users >24 weeks).[7]

The expectation that closed loop technology might offer something additional to existing delivery systems during pregnancy was examined in a recent open-label, crossover study, which showed that 74.7% of women with overnight closed loop were in the target range (3.5–7.8 mmol/L) overnight compared with 59.5% with sensor-augmented pump therapy.[36] However, the time in target was much lower at 66.3% with closed loop versus 56.8% with sensor-augmented pump therapy when both day and night periods were included.

Continuous Glucose Monitoring Systems in Pregnancy

An RCT that compared CGMS with or without conventional glucose monitoring every 4 to 6 weeks between 8 and 32 weeks gestation in 46 type 1 and 25 type 2 women showed an improvement in mean HbA1c in late pregnancy (5.8% vs 6.4%; $P = .0007$), with lower LGA rates (35% vs 60%) compared with conventional monitoring.[37] A subsequent Danish RCT of intermittent real-time CGM (RT-CGM) versus self-monitored plasma glucose 7 times daily showed no improvement in glycemic control or pregnancy outcome in women with pregestational diabetes, although women were tightly controlled at conception (HbA1c 6.6% vs 6.8% [49 vs 51 mmol/mol]), and in 60% use of RT-CGM was intermittent.[38]

A recent multicenter trial (CONCEPTT)[39] of women with T1DM showed that pregnant women randomized to RT-CGM had a reduction in HbA1c (0.19%; 95% $P = .0207$), more time in target (68% vs 61%; $P = .00344$), and less time hyperglycemic (27% vs 32%; $P = .0279$) than pregnant control participants, although with no difference in severe hypoglycemic episodes. In addition, with RT-CGM there was a lower incidence of LGA (odds ratio = 0.51; $P = .0210$), fewer neonatal intensive care admissions lasting more than 24 hours (0.48; 0.26–0.86; $P = .0157$), fewer incidences of neonatal hypoglycemia (0.45; 0.22–0.89; $P = .0250$), and 1-day shorter length of hospital stay (P = .0091). There was no apparent benefit of CGM in women planning pregnancy.

The CONCEPTT trial would support a role for CGMS in the management of pregnant women with T1DM, possibly in preference to CSII, given the lack of difference between CSII and MDI groups. Trials are now in progress to evaluate closed loop insulin delivery systems compared with conventional methods; however, preliminary data suggest that daytime in target is no greater with these devices than with CGMS, and greater emphasis may be needed on very fast-acting insulin analogs to reduce postprandial glucose excursions. Adverse reactions (particular skin) from CGMS devices are high, and may limit usage or even reliability of readings.[40] There is also a need for universal agreement regarding CGMS metrics, including time in target goals, nocturnal glucose ranges, expression of postprandial spikes, and the threshold for hypoglycemia during pregnancy. Universally, the cost of this technology is likely to restrict its use to selected, educated, motivated women in experienced centers receiving dedicated supervision.

OBSTETRIC SURVEILLANCE

Accurate dating of the pregnancy is an imperative, and is best achieved by ultrasound examination at 8 to 10 weeks. The goal of obstetric surveillance is to identify the fetus at risk, and to intervene in a timely and appropriate fashion to reduce perinatal morbidity and mortality.

Fetal monitoring in women with diabetes is as per routine antenatal care and includes a 20-week anomaly scan and fetal cardiac scan. The UK guideline[21] recommends ultrasound monitoring of fetal growth and amniotic fluid volume every 4 weeks from 28 to 36 weeks, and individualized monitoring of fetal wellbeing for women at risk of intrauterine growth restriction (IUGR), those with macrovascular disease, or those with nephropathy. Tests of fetal wellbeing before 38 weeks are not recommended unless there is a risk of IUGR.

LABOR AND DELIVERY

The primary objectives are to avoid fetal death in utero and the hazards of obstructed labor or shoulder dystocia associated with fetal macrosomia. As a consequence, caesarean section rates for women with pregestational diabetes in most parts of the world are over 50% (65% in the 2016 UK National Diabetes in Pregnancy Audit).[7] Iatrogenic prematurity has resulted in high rates of admission to NICU in T1DM.

Given the increased risk of preterm delivery, LGA, and perinatal mortality, close surveillance of mother and baby by an experienced obstetrician is needed during delivery. The timing and mode of birth should be discussed with the woman during her antenatal appointments. An individualized approach is required with particular consideration to fetal wellbeing, estimated size, glycemic control, diabetes complications, and past obstetric history.

UK NICE guidelines advise that women with T1DM should be offered an elective delivery between 37^{+0} and 38^{+6} weeks gestation, assuming no other significant factors have developed before this time.[21] An elective birth before 37^{+0} weeks should be considered if significant metabolic or any other maternal or fetal complications occur.

Preterm labor can be particularly hazardous for the infant of the diabetic mother. Beta-sympathomimetics agents used to suppress uterine contractions, and corticosteroids used to accelerate fetal lung maturation, may result in significant and prolonged maternal hyperglycemia, and even ketoacidosis, and the need for supplementary insulin must be anticipated. Several algorithms to guide glycemic management during steroid therapy have been developed.[23] Admission to hospital and close supervision is essential.

The management of labor should follow standard practice, as for nondiabetic women. Given the desire not to prolong pregnancy unduly, induction of labor is widely used, and usually involves prostaglandins, followed frequently by oxytocin. Careful monitoring of progress is facilitated by a partograph and continuous electronic fetal monitoring by cardiotocography.

Management of diabetes during labor should follow an established protocol, adapted for time and mode of delivery, in a dedicated center with a neonatal care unit equipped and staffed to deliver the most sophisticated level of care (exemplified in **Box 3**). Women with T1DM who use CSII should have the opportunity to discuss glycemic management during labor, in advance of delivery, with their physician, and an individualized plan should be clearly documented in their chart. UK NICE guidelines recommend maintenance of maternal blood glucose between 4 and 7 mmol/L during labor and delivery to reduce the incidence of neonatal hypoglycemia and fetal distress.[21,23] Hourly capillary glucose measurements provide a ready guide to the success of management and the need for insulin adjustment. Commonly used regimens (in the absence of a consensus) involve a constant glucose infusion, with insulin being infused separately by an infusion pump.[21,23] It is essential that, whatever regimen is used, midwifery and anesthetic staff are familiar with it.

Box 3
Intra-delivery protocol and method of delivery

Elective caesarean section

- Women with type 1 diabetes should be placed first on the operating list and admitted either the previous day or early on the morning of surgery
- Long-acting insulin is taken as normal before a light supper
- The mother should fast from 22:00 h the evening before surgery and should be first on the operating list the next day; rapid-acting insulin should be withheld
- 1 to 2 hours before surgery, hourly monitoring of blood glucose begins; and a glucose-insulin infusion is commenced, if necessary, to maintain blood glucose between 4 and 7 mmol/L
- The insulin dose and/or rate is adjusted in response to maternal/capillary glucose

Induction of labor

- Women should continue their current insulin regimen until labor is confirmed
- Often, an early morning breakfast is consumed with their normal morning insulin dose
- Once labor is confirmed and mother is fasting, glucose-insulin infusion is commenced as per protocol, unless delivery is imminent
- Maternal blood glucose levels should be monitored hourly
- Blood glucose levels should be maintained between 4 and 7 mmol/L
- The insulin dose/and or rate is adjusted in response to maternal blood glucose

Spontaneous labor

- Following admission in spontaneous labor, the patient is fasted
- A blood glucose level should be taken on admission and hourly thereafter
- Once labor is confirmed, a glucose-insulin infusion is commenced as per protocol
- Capillary glucose levels should be maintained between 4 and 7 mmol/L
- The insulin dose and/or rate is adjusted according to the local protocol in response to maternal blood glucose

MANAGEMENT OF DIABETES POSTPARTUM

Insulin sensitivity increases in the immediate postpartum period, normalizing over the following 1 to 2 weeks. Once the cord is cut, an insulin infusion should be reduced by 50%, with regular capillary blood glucose measurement and administration of IV fluids until the mother is eating normally. This should be done with close supervision by the diabetes care team, and insulin titration as required. Mothers with diabetes are encouraged to eat a small snack before breastfeeding to avoid hypoglycemia. Insulin requirements may increase during the day owing to increased caloric intake, with a fall in nocturnal insulin requirements owing to glucose siphoning into the breast milk. Women are therefore advised to reduce their long-acting insulin when breastfeeding. Maternal glucose should be kept as normal as possible to avoid elevations in milk glucose and maternal hypoglycemia. This is achieved through regular snacking and careful insulin adjustment, with full support from the diabetes specialist team.

NEONATAL CARE

Neonates born to women with T1DM should have their blood glucose measured using a method validated for neonatal use. Women should feed their babies within 30 minutes of birth and then at frequent intervals (every 2–3 hours) until feeding maintains prefeeding capillary plasma glucose levels at a minimum of 2.0 mmol/L. If capillary plasma glucose values are below 2.0 mmol/L on 2 consecutive readings, despite maximal support for feeding, or if there are abnormal clinical signs, or if the baby will not feed orally effectively, additional measures such as tube feeding or intravenous dextrose should be used. Up to 50% of babies may need to be admitted to neonatal intensive care[41] for the following indications (**Box 4**):

Neonates should not be transferred to community care until they are at least 24 hours old and are maintaining their blood glucose at a normal level and feeding well.

Box 4
Indications for admission to neonatal intensive care

- Hypoglycemia associated with abnormal clinical signs respiratory distress
- Signs of cardiac decompensation from congenital heart disease or cardiomyopathy
- Signs of neonatal encephalopathy
- Signs of polycythemia and are likely to need partial exchange transfusion
- Need for intravenous fluids
- Tube feeding (unless adequate support is available on the postnatal ward)
- Jaundice requiring intense phototherapy and frequent monitoring of bilirubinemia
- Delivery before 34 weeks (or between 34 and 36 weeks if dictated clinically by the initial assessment of the baby and feeding on the labor ward)

POSTPARTUM CONTRACEPTION

As mentioned earlier, it is of vital importance that women with T1DM plan their pregnancy to optimize their glucose control. Selection of a method of contraception should consider the following:

- The method should be effective; an unplanned pregnancy in this population group is associated with an increased risk for many maternal and neonatal outcomes

- The method should not affect insulin sensitivity or glucose metabolism
- Contraception should not interfere with breast feeding or increase the risk of postpartum depressive disorders
- It should be convenient to use
- It should be safe to use with the presence of existing comorbidities
- It should not increase long-term cardiovascular risk factors, such as those associated with diabetic complications

There is a growing opinion that suggests that contraception should be initiated before the woman is discharged from hospital. This is because of the recognition that ovulation and sexual activity occurs much earlier than previously estimated.[42] In addition, many women miss their postpartum appointments. The World Health Organization has stated that virtually all methods of contraception can be offered to women with T1DM.[43] However, estrogen-containing methods should be avoided by women with diabetic complications for example, retinopathy, nephropathy, or cardiovascular disease. Intrauterine contraceptive methods are particularly suited to women who do not wish to become pregnant within the next year. In women without vascular disease who wish to conceive sooner, combined (estrogen and progesterone) hormonal contraception is considered safe. The lowest dose (estrogen <35 mg) and potency formulation should be used, as here the absolute increase in arterial thromboembolism is very low (1/12,000) and comparable with that among healthy users and nonusers. Barrier and natural family planning methods are less ideal because of high failure rates. Following completion of childbearing, vasectomy and female sterilization are available.

Women with T1DM should revert to their routine diabetes care under the supervision of their diabetes care team. Women planning further pregnancies should be reminded of the need for preconception planning for an optimum pregnancy outcome (**Box 5**).

Box 5
Future challenges and possible solutions

- Despite modern obstetric and neonatal care, type 1 diabetes remains a high risk situation for mother and baby.

- Encouraging women to plan their pregnancy is a major challenge and can only be addressed by a multilayered approach, including harnessing public and professional methods to increase awareness beginning in adolescence, maximizing family doctor and pharmacist points of contact, sensitive timely contraceptive advice, and judicious use of social media.

- Multidisciplinary team working in the same geographic setting is a recommended model that provides coherence of care.

- There is a need for better methods to identify women at increased risk of fetal compromise toward the end of pregnancy for whom early delivery is indicated.

- It is likely that the next decade will have an increasing technological focus but detailed evaluation is required of the relative roles of CGM, CSII/RT-CGMS, and closed loop devices, together with rapid-acting insulin analogs in optimizing glycemic control in selected patients.

REFERENCES

1. International Diabetes Federational. IDF Atlas. 8th Edition 2017. Available at: https://diabetesatlas.org/resources/2017-atlas.html. Accessed June 14, 2019.

2. The Healthcare Quality Improvement Partnership. National pregnancy in diabetes audit report, 2015. 2016. Available at: https://www.hqip.org.uk/search/?fwp_

resources_search=national pregnancy in diabetes audit 2015 2016#.XQU7h 7mWwdU. Accessed June 14, 2019.

3. Mayer-Davis EJ, Bell RA, Dabelea D, et al. SEARCH for Diabetes in Youth Study Group. The many faces of diabetes in American youth: type 1 and type 2 diabetes in five race and ethnic populations: the SEARCH for Diabetes in Youth Study. Diabetes Care 2009;32(Supplement 2):S99–101.

4. Lin Y, Chen K, Peng Y, et al. Type 1 diabetes impairs female fertility even before it is diagnosed. Diabetes Res Clin Pract 2018;143:151–8.

5. Colstrup M, Mathiesen ER, Damm P, et al. Pregnancy in women with type 1 diabetes: Have the goals of St. Vincent declaration been met concerning foetal and neonatal complications? J Matern Fetal Neonatal Med 2013;26(17):1682–6.

6. CEMACH. Confidential Enquiry into maternal and Child health (CEMACH), pregnancy in women with type 1 and type 2 diabetes in 2002-2003, England, Wales and Northern Ireland. London. 2005. Available at: https://elearning.rcog.org.uk//sites/default/files/Diabetes%20and%20other%20endocrinopathies/CEMACH_Pregnancy_type_1_2_diabetes.pdf. Accessed June 14, 2019.

7. UK National Diabetes in Pregnancy Audit. 2016. Available at: https://digital.nhs.uk/data-and-information/publications/statistical/national-pregnancy-in-diabetes-audit/national-pregnancy-in-diabetes-annual-report-2016. Accessed June 14, 2019.

8. Felig P, Lynch V. Starvation in human pregnancy: hypoglycaemia, hypoinsulinaemia and hyperketonaemia. Science 1970;170:990–2.

9. Catalano PM, Tyzbir ED, Wolfe RR, et al. Longitudinal changes in basal hepatic glucose production and suppression during insulin infusion in normal pregnant women. Am J Obstet Gynecol 1992;167(4 Pt 1):913–9.

10. Freemark M. Regulation of maternal metabolism by pituitary and placental hormones: roles in fetal development and metabolic programming. Horm Res 2006;65(Suppl 3):41–9.

11. Ray JG, O'Brien TE, Chan WS. Preconception care and the risk of congenital anomalies in offspring of women with diabetes mellitus: a meta-analysis. QJM 2001;9:435–44.

12. Wahabi HA, Alzeidan RA, Esmaeil SA. Pre-pregnancy care for women with pre-gestational diabetes mellitus: a systematic review and meta-analysis. BMC Public Health 2012;12:792.

13. Bell K, Glinianaia S, Tennant P, et al. Peri-conception hyperglycaemia and nephropathy are associated with risk of congenital anomaly in women with pre-existing diabetes: a population-based cohort study. Diabetologia 2012;55:936–47.

14. Temple RC, Stanley KP. Pre-pregnancy care in type 1 and type 2 diabetes. In: McCance DR, Maresh M, Sacks DA, editors. A practical manual of diabetes in pregnancy. 2nd edition. Oxford (United Kingdom): Wiley Blackwell; 2018. p. 129–39.

15. Morrison M, Hendrieckx C, Nankervis A, et al. Factors associated with attendance for pre-pregnancy care and reasons for non-attendance among women with diabetes. Diabetes Res Clin Pract 2018;142:269–75.

16. Murphy HR, Temple RC, Ball VE, et al. Personal experiences of women with diabetes who do not attend pre-pregnancy care. Diabet Med 2010;27(1):92–100.

17. Ringholm L, Pedersen-Bjergaard U, Thorsteinsson B, et al. Hypoglycaemia during pregnancy in women with type 1 diabetes. Diabet Med 2012;29(5):558–66.

18. Rizzo T, Metzger BE, Burns WJ, et al. Correlations between antepartum maternal metabolism and intelligence of offspring. N Engl J Med 1991;325(13):911–6.

19. Sahaipal NS, Goel RK, Chaubey A, et al. Pathological perturbations in diabetic retinopathy: hyperglycemia, AGEs, oxidative stress and inflammatory pathways. Curr Protein Pept Sci 2019;20(1):92–119.

20. Hasan J, Chew EY. Retinopathy in diabetic pregnancy. In: McCance DR, Maresh M, Sacks DA, editors. Practical manual of diabetes in pregnancy. Blackwell-Wiley; 2018. p. 269–83.

21. National Institute for Health and Care Excellence. Diabetes in pregnancy: management from preconception to the postnatal period 2015. Available at: https://www.nice.org.uk/guidance/ng3/resources/diabetes-in-pregnancy-management-from-preconception-to-the-postnatal-period-pdf-51038446021. Accessed June 14, 2019.

22. Mathiesen ER, Ringholm L, Damm P. Complications in pregnancy: hypertension and diabetic nephropathy in diabetes in pregnancy. In: McCance DR, Maresh M, Sacks DA, editors. Practical manual of diabetes in pregnancy. Blackwell-Wiley; 2010. p. 257–68.

23. Management of glycaemic control in pregnant women with diabetes. Available at: http://www.diabetologists-abcd.org.uk/JBDS/JBDS_Pregnancy_201017.pdf. Accessed June 14, 2019.

24. American Diabetes Association. Management of diabetes in pregnancy: standards of medical care in diabetes- 2018. Diabetes Care 2018;41(1):137–43.

25. Maresh MJ, Holmes VA, Patterson CC, et al. Glycemic targets in the second and third trimester of pregnancy for women with type 1 diabetes. Diabetes Care 2015; 38:34–42.

26. Holmes VA, Young IS, Patterson CC, et al. Optimal glycemic control, preeclampsia, and gestational hypertension in women with type 1 diabetes in the diabetes and pre-eclampsia intervention trial. Diabetes Care 2011;34:683–8.

27. Pickup JC, Freeman SC, Sutton AJ. Glycaemic control in type 1 diabetes during real time continuous glucose monitoring compared with self monitoring of blood glucose: meta-analysis of randomised controlled trials using individual patient data. BMJ 2011;343:d3805.

28. Kerssen A, Evers IM, Visser VH. Day to day glucose variability during pregnancy in women with type 1 diabetes mellitus: glucose profiles measured with the continuous glucose monitoring system. Br J Obstet Gynaecol 2004;111:919–24.

29. Wright LA, Hirsch IB. Metrics beyond haemoglobin A1c in diabetes management: time in range, hypoglycemia, and other parameters. Diabetes Technol Ther 2017; 19(2):s16–26.

30. Murphy HR, Rayman G, Duffield K, et al. Changes in the glycaemic profiles of women with type 1 and type 2 diabetes during pregnancy. Diabetes Care 2007;30:2785–91.

31. Manderson JG, Patterson CC, Hadden DR, et al. Preprandial versus postprandial blood glucose monitoring in type 1 diabetic pregnancy: a randomized controlled clinical trial. Am J Obstet Gynecol 2003;189:507–12.

32. Damm P, Mersebach H, Råstam J, et al. Poor pregnancy outcome in women with type 1 diabetes is predicted by elevated HbA1c and spikes of high glucose values in the third trimester. J Matern Fetal Neonatal Med 2014;27(2):149–54.

33. Mathiesen ER, Damm P, Hod M, et al. Maternal glycaemic control and hypoglycaemia in type 1 diabetic pregnancy: a randomised trial of insulin aspart versus human insulin in 322 pregnant women. Diabetes Care 2007;30:771–6.

34. Mathiesen ER, Hod M, Ivanisevic M, et al, on behalf of the Detemir in Pregnancy Study Group. Maternal efficacy and safety outcomes in a randomized, controlled

trial comparing insulin detemir with NPH insulin in 310 pregnant women with type 1 diabetes. Diabetes Care 2012;35(10):2012–7.

35. Cummins E, Royle P, Snaith A, et al. Clinical effectiveness and cost-effectiveness of continuous subcutaneous insulin infusion for diabetes: a systematic review and economic evaluation. Health Technol Assess 2010;11:1–181.

36. Stewart ZA, Wilinska ME, Hartnell S, et al. Closed-loop insulin delivery during pregnancy in women with type 1 diabetes. N Engl J Med 2016;375:644–54.

37. Murphy HR, Rayman G, Lewis K, et al. Effectiveness of continuous glucose monitoring in pregnant women with diabetes: randomized clinical trial. BMJ 2008;337:2003–15.

38. Secher AL, Ringholm L, Andersen HU, et al. The effect of real-time continuous glucose monitoring in pregnant women with diabetes: a randomised controlled clinical trial. Diabetes Care 2013;36:1877–83.

39. Feig DS, Donovan LE, Corcoy R, et al. Continuous glucose monitoring in pregnant women with type 1 diabetes (CONCEPTT): a multicentre international randomised controlled trial. Lancet 2017;390(10110):2347–59.

40. Bolinder J, Antuna R, Geelhoed-Duijvestijn P, et al. Novel sensing technology and hypoglycaemia in type 1 diabetes: a multicentre, non-masked, randomised controlled trial. Lancet 2016;388:2254–63.

41. McCance DR, Holmes VA, Maresh MJ, et al. Vitamins C and E for prevention of pre-eclampsia in women with type 1 diabetes (DAPIT): a randomised placebo-controlled trial. Lancet 2010;376(9737):259–66.

42. Jackson E, Glasier A. Return of ovulation and menses in postpartum nonlactating women. Obstet Gynecol 2011;117:657–62.

43. World Health Organization. Medical eligibility criteria for contraceptive use, 5th edition. Geneva (Switzerland). 2015. Available at: https://www.who.int/repro ductivehealth/publications/family_planning/Ex-Summ-MEC-5/en/. Accessed June 14, 2019.

Type 2 Diabetes in Pregnancy

Anil Kapur, MD[a,b,*], Harold David McIntyre, MD, FRACP[b,c],
Moshe Hod, MD[b,d]

KEYWORDS

- Pregnancy hyperglycemia • Type 2 diabetes • Management

KEY POINTS

- Hyperglycemia including previously unknown type 2 diabetes mellitus (DM) is a common medical condition during pregnancy, necessitating universal testing of all pregnant women including first trimester testing.
- Pregnancy-induced metabolic changes in women with type 2 DM require more intensive monitoring and closer titration of treatment to ensure glycemic control is optimized very early in pregnancy to reduce risk of fetal hyperinsulinemia.
- Women with type 2 DM have similar rates of major congenital malformations, stillbirth, and neonatal mortality, as seen in women with type 1 DM, but have a higher risk of perinatal mortality.
- In utero type 2 DM exposure confers greater risk and reduces time to development of type 2 DM in offspring compared with GDM and no diabetes exposure.
- Preconception care to improve metabolic control in women with type 2 DM is critical in improving outcome.

INTRODUCTION

Diabetes mellitus is rapidly escalating, with prevalence rates rising among all age groups. The International Diabetes Federation (IDF) estimates that diabetes affects about 415 million people globally and is projected to increase to 642 million people by 2040. There is an equally high burden of prediabetes—approximately 318 million, likely to increase to about 481 million by 2040.[1]

The prevalence of hyperglycemia in pregnancy (HIP) parallels the prevalence of prediabetes, type 2 diabetes (type 2 DM), and overweight and obesity in a given

Disclosure: The authors have nothing to disclose.
[a] World Diabetes Foundation, 30 A, Krogshoejvej, Bagsverd 2880, Denmark; [b] FIGO Pregnancy and NCD Committee, Jabotinski Street, Petah Tiqwa 49100, Israel; [c] UQ Mater Clinical Unit, Faculty of Medicine, Mater Health Services, University of Queensland, Raymond Terrace, South Brisbane, Brisbane, Qld 4101, Australia; [d] Department of Obstetrics and Gynecology, Clalit Health Services, Mor Women's Health Center, Rabin Medical Center, Tel Aviv University, 18 Aba Ahimeir St., Tel Aviv 6949204, Israel
* Corresponding author.
E-mail address: dr.anilkapur@gmail.com

Endocrinol Metab Clin N Am 48 (2019) 511–531
https://doi.org/10.1016/j.ecl.2019.05.009
0889-8529/19/© 2019 Elsevier Inc. All rights reserved.

population. In the absence of any symptoms more than half of people with type 2 DM, particularly the young and women, remain unaware and undiagnosed.[1] These conditions are increasingly affecting younger people in the reproductive age, thus more women entering pregnancy are vulnerable to HIP. The World Health Organization's (WHO) 2014 data,[2] showing that more than half of the world's adult population was overweight (39%) or obese (13%), including an estimated 42 million pregnant women, has important ramifications for the future burden of HIP, type 2 DM, obesity, and cardiovascular diseases.

Between 1994 and 2004, rates of type 2 DM in pregnancy increased by 347% in the United States.[3] Age-standardized prevalence of pre-pregnancy diabetes (PDM) increased by 37% (P<.01) in all age, race, and ethnicity groups, between 2000 and 2010.[4] In Scotland, between April 1998 and March 2013, the number of pregnancies complicated by type 2 DM increased by 90%.[5] In the United Kingdom, the prevalence of PDM increased by almost 50% between 1996 and 1998 and 2002 to 2004, driven mainly by an increase in type 2 DM.[6] Similarly, in Sweden between 1998 and 2012, and in Canada between 2002/2003 and 2011/2012, the number of pregnancies complicated by type 2 DM increased by 111%[7] and 250%,[8] respectively.

Reliable nationwide data from populous countries such as China and India are not available, but it is believed that the rates of type 2 DM in pregnancy are also rising significantly in these countries. A population study involving 2.1 million women planning pregnancy in China,[9] using fasting capillary plasma glucose, estimated diabetes and prediabetes prevalence of 1.4% and 12.9%, respectively. A study from Tamil Nadu, India, reported an overall prevalence of 2.6% for diabetes in pregnancy (DIP), presumed mostly to be type 2 DM; in the urban area the reported rate for DIP was as high as 7.7%.[10]

IDF estimates that 1 in 6 live births (16.8%) occur to women with some form of HIP, with 2.5% owing to overt DIP, with the remaining 14.3% (1 in 7 pregnancies) because of gestational diabetes mellitus (GDM).[1]

HYPERGLYCEMIA IN PREGNANCY: CLASSIFICATION

HIP is classified as either previously known type 1 DM or type 2 DM predating pregnancy; or hyperglycemia first detected during pregnancy. Depending on the glucose level, hyperglycemia, first detected at any time during pregnancy, is classified either as DIP or GDM. Women are considered to have overt diabetes or DIP if their plasma glucose values during pregnancy are above the WHO thresholds that define diabetes outside of pregnancy.[11] In the absence of ketoacidosis, or other evidence suggesting type 1 DM, such cases are assumed to have type 2 DM. Some of them, however, may be secondary to other pathologies (eg, pancreatic disease) or monogenic causes, collectively termed maturity onset diabetes of the young (MODY)—a group of autosomal dominant disorders caused by specific single-gene mutations. MODY accounts for less than 5% of diabetes; because of its rarity and phenotypic overlap with type 1 DM and type 2 DM, low awareness, and lack of diagnostic facilities it is often misdiagnosed.[12–14] Fourteen specific gene mutations have been identified,[15] of which 3 are responsible for 85% cases of MODY.

Prevalence of MODY in pregnancy is not well studied on a population basis. In carefully phenotypically selected women with fasting HIP 12 out of the 15 women screened had glucokinase gene mutations.[16] A study from India[17] reported that 18% women with HIP (5 PDM and 4 DIP) with a dominant family history of diabetes, carefully selected for screening, tested positive for MODY. Properly identifying MODY subtypes among women with HIP has relevance for clinical management.

PREGNANCY-INDUCED METABOLIC CHANGES AND DIABETES CONTROL

The feto-placental unit implants in the mother's uterus and grows until delivery. This is achieved through orchestrated multisystem adaptations in maternal physiology, including immunologic, endocrine and metabolic, cardiovascular, musculoskeletal, and respiratory system adaptations throughout pregnancy. These adaptations are modulated by complex interactions of the feto-placental-maternal unit to achieve a healthy balance between the mother's needs and demand for fetal growth and development.[18]

Implantation and placentation in the first and early second trimester of pregnancy resembles "an open wound in the uterus" that requires a strong inflammatory response.[19] The blastocyst breaks through the epithelial lining of the uterus to implant; breaches the endometrial lining to invade; followed by trophoblast replacement of the endothelium and vascular smooth muscle of the maternal blood vessels to secure an adequate placental-fetal blood supply. These activities create a veritable "battleground" of invading, dying, and repairing cells. An inflammatory environment is required to secure adequate repair of the uterine epithelium and removal of cellular debris.[20] High levels of the proinflammatory T helper 1 and cytokines (interleukin-6 [IL-6], IL-8, and tumor necrosis factor [TNF-α]) characterize early implantation. During most of the second and mid-third trimester, the mother, the placenta and the fetus are in a symbiotic relationship marked by state of immune tolerance to permit rapid fetal growth and development. Late third trimester and delivery is again marked by a proinflammatory response[21] with metabolic consequences. The proinflammatory environment promotes uterine contractions, leading to delivery of the baby and the placenta.

These inflammatory changes have endocrine consequences. Production of inflammatory mediators by the placenta—TNF-α and cytokines IL-6 and IL-8, and similar changes in the maternal adipose tissues—contribute to increasing insulin resistance.

Soon after implantation and placentation, circulating levels of human placental lactogen (hPL), placental growth hormone, progesterone, cortisol, prolactin, and other hormones increase, and contribute to increasing insulin resistance in maternal peripheral tissues throughout pregnancy.[22] The levels of the adipocyte- and increasingly placental-derived hormone leptin increase during late gestation and levels of adiponectin decline. To compensate for this, in normal nondiabetic pregnancies, circulating insulin levels and glucose-stimulated insulin secretory capacity of pancreatic β cells increase as gestation progresses. Increasing levels of prolactin and hPL enhance insulin secretion and also increase the size and number of pancreatic β cells.[23] MicroRNAs, specifically miR-338-3p, regulated by hormones including estradiol, may play a role in regulating β cell mass and function during pregnancy.[24] The role of incretins in enhancing insulin secretion and β cell mass during pregnancy is postulated but needs confirmation. The increased insulin resistance and the need for β cell adaptation to deal with it makes even a normal pregnancy a potent "metabolic stressor."[25–27]

In women with type 2 DM, pregnancy-induced insulin resistance adds to the preexisting insulin resistance, and the preexisting pancreatic β cell defect compromises the ability to enhance insulin secretion during pregnancy, leading to marked hyperglycemia.

Pregnancy-induced metabolic changes in women with type 2 DM require more intensive monitoring and closer titration of treatment. In normal pregnancy in the first trimester, as maternal plasma volume increases, fasting plasma glucose declines because of the dilution effect. In pregnant women with type 2 DM this decline may be blunted. During the second and third trimesters, the normal increase in hepatic gluconeogenesis and lipolysis is further enhanced in women with type 2 DM, and postprandial suppression of hepatic gluconeogenesis may not occur. Coupled with reduced peripheral glucose uptake, this causes higher postprandial glucose spikes. Significant changes in protein and lipid metabolism are also seen.[28]

Placental and fetal uptake of glucose are also important variables affecting maternal glucose levels. Fetal hyperinsulinemia increases fetal glucose use, and, by lowering fetal glycaemia, increases the glucose concentration gradient across the placenta, increasing glucose flux to the fetus. This helps to lower maternal glucose level, favoring a persistently high glucose flux, even when maternal blood glucose is not very high. This is called the "fetal glucose steal" syndrome, in which a hyperinsulinemic macrosomic fetus apparently helps to attenuate and "normalize" maternal glucose despite poor maternal metabolic control. This provides an explanation for why some mothers with fetuses with all the characteristics of diabetic fetopathy have apparently "good" glucose control.[29]

The obvious implication is that glycemic control needs to be optimized very early in pregnancy to prevent the establishment of fetal hyperinsulinemia, reinforcing the critical importance of pre-pregnancy planning and early establishment of maternal glycemic control.

CONSEQUENCES OF TYPE 2 DIABETES IN PREGNANCY

The association between maternal plasma glucose and adverse pregnancy outcomes is linear and continuous with no inflection point.[30] The quantum of hyperglycemic exposure in terms of duration and degree are relevant, as is the timing of the onset of exposure in the course of pregnancy. Early exposure during fetal organogenesis and placental development has more severe and lasting consequences then later exposure.

The abnormal metabolic environment of the mother with DM affects the developing fetal tissues, organs, and control systems in complex ways, which eventually lead to permanent functional changes in adult life.[31] Exposure to an abnormal mixture of metabolites may modify the phenotypic expression of the newly formed cells, which will in turn determine either the permanent, or short-term and long-term effects on the offspring. Depending on the timing of exposure to the aberrant fuel mixture (embryonic-fetal), different effects may occur.

Previously unknown diabetes at conception and embryogenesis increases the vulnerability to complications, in particular disrupted organogenesis with high risks of spontaneous abortion and congenital anomalies. Because of its earlier presence and greater hyperglycemia, DIP may cause more severe macrosomia by the earlier and more intense priming of the fetal β cell mass and persistence of fetal hyperinsulinemia throughout pregnancy, even when the mother enjoys good metabolic control in later pregnancy.[32,33] Conversely, through its effect on poor placentation, intrauterine growth restriction may result. PDM (both type 1 and 2) is associated with small-for- and large-for-gestational age placentas, respectively, in nearly 20% and 30% pregnancies.

Both type 1 DM and type 2 DM share similar incidences of preeclampsia and significant placental pathology; however, maternal decidual vasculopathy and reduced placental size (fetal-to-placental weight ratio <10th percentile) are more in women with type 2 DM.[34] The consequent placental dysfunction may turn the placenta from a "fetus protector" to a potential source of damaging outcomes.[35] The impact of maternal hyperglycemia on the fetus and perinatal outcomes is a sum total of the complex interplay of multiple variables.

Type 2 DM in pregnancy carries risks of adverse perinatal outcomes at least as severe as in type 1 DM. A systematic review and metaanalysis of 33 eligible studies reported that, despite lower glycated hemoglobin (HbA1c) at booking and throughout pregnancy, women with type 2 DM had a higher risk of perinatal mortality, less diabetic ketoacidosis and cesarean sections, and similar rates of major congenital malformations, stillbirth, and neonatal mortality, compared with type 1 DM.[36] Hyperglycemia significantly increases the risk of pregnancy complications (**Box 1**).[37,38] The risk, severity, and number of complications are directly related to level of maternal hyperglycemia and the stage of pregnancy at which exposure starts.

Box 1
Maternal and fetal morbidity associated with type 2 DM in pregnancy

Maternal
- Pre- and early pregnancy
  ○ Failure to conceive
  ○ Repeated spontaneous abortions
- During pregnancy
  ○ Preeclampsia
  ○ Gestational hypertension
  ○ Excessive fetal growth (macrosomia, large for gestational age)
  ○ Fetal growth restriction (intrauterine growth restriction, small for gestational age)
  ○ Polyhydramnios
  ○ Urinary tract infections
  ○ Labile/worsening glucose control
  ○ Progression/new onset diabetic retinopathy
  ○ Worsening of preexisting renal disease
  ○ Preterm labor
- During labor and delivery
  ○ Traumatic labor
  ○ Shoulder dystocia
  ○ Instrumental delivery
  ○ Cesarean delivery
  ○ Postoperative/postpartum hemorrhage
  ○ Thromboembolism
  ○ Maternal mortality
- Puerperium
  ○ Failure to initiate and/or maintain breast feeding
  ○ Postoperative/postpartum infection
- Long-term postpartum
  ○ Weight retention
  ○ Worsening glucose control
  ○ Future cardiovascular disease

Fetal/neonatal
- Stillbirth
- Neonatal death
- Nonchromosomal congenital malformations
- Respiratory distress syndrome
- Cardiomyopathy
- Neonatal hypoglycemia
- Neonatal polycythemia
- Neonatal hyperbilirubinemia
- Neonatal hypocalcemia
- Programming and imprinting; fetal origins of disease: diabetes, obesity, hypertension
- Higher risk of attention-deficit hyperactivity disorders; autism spectrum disorders

Congenital anomalies are commonly reported in offspring of women with diabetes.[39,40] A Danish study reported an odds ratio of 2.1 (95% CI: 1.5–3.1) for congenital abnormalities in infants of women with diabetes, with particularly strong associations for renal agenesis, obstructive urinary tract anomalies, cardiovascular, and multiple congenital abnormalities.[39]

Between 2002/2003 and 2012/2013, the prevalence of congenital anomalies in Canada was approximately 42 per 1000 live births. Several specific congenital anomalies decreased; however, a significant increase in congenital anomalies linked to PDM was noted over the same time period. In 2012/2013, the rate of any congenital anomaly among women with PDM was 93.4 per 1000 live births, with no difference between type 1 DM and type 2 DM.[41] In the United States, the relative risks of stillbirth (2.51), miscarriage (1.28), and cesarean section (1.77) were significantly greater with type 2 DM versus nondiabetes[42]; 1 in 3 infants of mothers with type 2 DM require neonatal intensive care unit (NICU) admissions.[43] The problem of poor pregnancy outcome with type 2 DM is compounded in adolescent and very young pregnancies, in which 1 in 4 end in miscarriage, stillbirth, or intrauterine death; and 1 in 5 of the liveborn infants have a major congenital anomaly.[44]

Independent of genetic risk, offspring of hyperglycemic pregnancies are at increased risk of early onset type 2 DM and obesity. Important differences exist in offspring risk of diabetes based on type of diabetes exposure in utero. In utero type 2 DM exposure confers greater risk and reduces time to development of type 2 DM in offspring compared with GDM and no diabetes exposure.[45] Other studies have also reported significantly higher risk of type 2 DM in offspring of diabetic mothers.[46–48]

Although IQ scores of children born to well-controlled diabetic mothers are similar to those of control children, a negative correlation has been shown between severity of maternal hyperglycemia and performance on various neurodevelopmental and behavioral tests.[49] Compared with children unexposed to diabetes in utero, children exposed to diabetes have been reported to be at higher risks for attention-deficit hyperactivity disorders,[50] autism spectrum disorders, and intellectual disabilities.[51,52] A more marked effect has been reported with combined exposure to maternal prepregnancy obesity and diabetes.

Pregnancy increases the short-term risk of occurrence and progression of diabetic retinopathy[53–56]; progression occurs at approximately double the rate in pregnant women.[57] Progression is influenced by diabetes duration, glycemic control before and during pregnancy, pregnancy-induced hypertension, diabetic nephropathy, and preeclampsia.

Young people with type 2 DM have a similar[58] or higher prevalence of hypertension and microalbuminuria, and higher risk of renal failure,[59] compared with youth with type 1 DM.

Pregnancies in women with diabetic nephropathy are challenging, with outcomes worse than expected for the stage of kidney disease in women without diabetes. Maternal hypertension, preeclampsia, and cesarean section rates are high, and offspring are often preterm and of low birth weight.[60] With careful preconception assessment, optimized glycemic control, and adjustment of medical treatment, progression of nephropathy can be prevented and kidney function preserved.[61]

Maternal obesity and gestational weight gain have a significant impact on maternal metabolism and offspring development. Insulin resistance, glucose homeostasis, fat oxidation, and amino acid synthesis are all disrupted by maternal obesity and contribute to adverse outcomes.[28] Comorbid obesity adds further complexity to the metabolic conundrum of pre-pregnancy type 2 DM. Further discussion on this subject is beyond the scope of this paper.

Because undiagnosed type 2 DM in pregnancy has severe consequences for both the mother and the fetus, and has greater likelihood of occurrence because of the high rates of diabetes and risk factors in the background population, testing all pregnant women without known diabetes for hyperglycemia at first booking to rule out preexisting diabetes is now increasingly recommended and accepted.[62]

MANAGEMENT
Preconception Care and Pregnancy Planning

Management of reproductive-age women with diabetes needs substantial improvement.[63] Women with type 2 DM are at higher risk of adverse pregnancy outcomes associated with poor pregnancy preparation, even compared with women with type 1 DM, because they are less aware and less likely to access Pre-pregnancy care (PPC). Challenges and barriers include lack of time and awareness of the need for PPC; limited knowledge among primary health care professionals; limited access to specialist PPC[64]; complexity of care setting and infrequent consultations.[65] Women with type 2 DM remain less likely to take 5 mg preconception folic acid and more likely to take potentially harmful medications than women with type 1 DM.[66] There is a clear need to integrate reproductive health into diabetes care, improve uptake of prepregnancy and postnatal care to improve health outcomes of women with diabetes.[65,66]

Culturally appropriate, women-centered, community-based PPC programs can bring clinically relevant improvements to pregnancy preparation in women with type 2 DM[67] by changing the process of clinical care delivery and using evidence-based interventions in pragmatic clinical settings.[68] Targeted PPC for women with diabetes is cost saving.[69,70]

The key tasks pre-pregnancy care for women with type 2 DM are

1. *Medical and obstetric history review; assessment of physical and metabolic status and screening for complications and comorbid conditions.* A complete medical and obstetric history review including audit of current medications (both prescription and frequently used over-the-counter drugs) should be done. Particular attention should be paid to screen for comorbid hypertension, preexisting retinopathy, nephropathy, thyroid disorders, cardiac conditions, and presence of lurking infections, allergies, and drug sensitivities. The pre-pregnancy testing protocol should include tests for blood group, anemia, HbA1c, thyroid-stimulating hormone, dipstick for proteinuria, creatinine, and urinary albumin to creatinine ratio, rubella, syphilis, hepatitis B, HIV, Pap smear, and cervical culture.[71] Drugs with potentially harmful effects should be replaced with safe alternatives. In particular, medications for hypertension require review. Angiotensin receptor blockers and angiotensin-converting enzyme (ACE) inhibitors should be replaced[71] with alpha methyldopa, labetalol, nifedipine, or diltiazem; statins should be discontinued,[71] and guidance provided for use of pain medications, and so forth.

2. *Glycemic control before conception.* Glycemic targets should be set based on the above review in consultation with the patient and should aim to achieve glucose control as close to normal as possible. Pre-pregnancy glycemic control assessment should be based on HbA1c measurement and not merely relied on spot tests (fasting or postprandial measurement). Two consecutive HbA1c readings below 6.5%–7.0% measured 3 months apart before conception considerably improve chances of better outcome, provided good control is also maintained throughout

pregnancy. This requires intensification of medical treatment and greater attention to nutrition and physical activity. It may be preferable to shift to insulin treatment to achieve control when conception is planned.

3. *Maintain effective contraception until glycemic targets are achieved.* Women should receive advice and be offered safe and effective methods of contraception. Patients' preference, diabetes status, and presence of complications are significant determinants in selecting the contraceptive method. Although data are sparse, no worsening of glycemic control or on the course of microvascular complications has been reported in diabetic women with use of combined oral contraceptives (OCs).[72] Use of low-dose combined pills is now considered safe for women with uncomplicated diabetes but requires caution when used in the presence of associated cardiovascular risk or disease, or severe microvascular complications, such as nephropathy with proteinuria or active proliferative retinopathy.[72] Caution must also be used in prescribing combined hormonal contraception in obese women with type 2 DM. Progestin-only contraceptives, as well as nonhormonal methods, provide useful alternatives.[72] Long-acting reversible contraceptives (LARCs) are excellent choices for women with type 2 DM.[73] LARCs include intrauterine devices and implants. LARC methods are highly effective, with no patient adherence issues. Even though up-front costs are higher, LARCs are among the most cost-effective contraception available because of their low failure rate. Pregnancy may occur soon after discontinuation of OCs and it is advisable to advise use of other methods for a short time after OC discontinuation to allow clearance from the body before conception.

4. *Supplement folic acid.* Treat anemia and other nutritional deficiencies, in particular, vitamin D and calcium, if present.

5. *Initiate lifestyle changes and weight control measures.* Pre-pregnancy is the ideal time to initiate lifestyle counseling in general, including advice on healthy eating, exercise, smoking cessation, and guidance on alcohol consumption and exposure to harmful environmental pollutants, including certain personal care products to reduce exposure to endocrine-disrupting chemicals. Overweight and obese women should be encouraged to lose weight to reduce risk of complications.

MANAGEMENT OF TYPE 2 DIABETES DURING PREGNANCY
Monitoring—Glucose and Microvascular Complications

Maternal and fetal outcomes in women with type 2 DM are directly correlated with the degree of glycemic control. The primary goal of treatment is to ensure as close to normal glucose values as possible, such that the developing fetus has minimal exposure to hyperglycemia.

Blood glucose control can be evaluated in 1 of 3 ways: HbA1c, self-monitoring of blood glucose (SMBG), and continuous glucose monitoring (CGM).

- *HbA1c:* best used during PPC and in antenatal follow-up of PDM or DIP. The HbA1c-average glucose relationship is altered by pregnancy; therefore it is not a reliable marker for diabetes control during pregnancy and must be supplemented with other measures.
- *SMBG:* is recommended as a key component of the management plan for diabetes during pregnancy. The usefulness of SMBG in helping achieve glycemic control to reduce pregnancy complications is well recognized.[74] There is no evidence that any specific glucose monitoring protocol or technique is superior to any other technique among pregnant women with preexisting type 1 DM or type 2 DM.[75]

- *CGM:* use has been shown to improve control in people with diabetes. It is particularly useful in detecting high postprandial glucose levels and nocturnal hypoglycemia. CGM provides detailed information concerning glycemic fluctuations.[76–78] The recently published CONCEPTT trial has demonstrated improved outcomes with CGM in women with type 1 DM, but clear evidence is lacking in type 2 DM.[79]

There is insufficient evidence concerning the optimal frequency of blood glucose testing for pregnant women with type 2 DM.[75] In its 2018 clinical practice recommendations, the American Diabetes Association (ADA) encourages preprandial and postprandial monitoring of blood glucose, but does not recommend a specific frequency of testing.[71] The International Federation of Gynecology and Obstetrics (FIGO) made recommendations for glucose monitoring based on resource settings (**Table 1**).[62]

Women with type 2 DM previously not assessed before pregnancy, or those diagnosed with DIP on routine testing, must undergo tests to rule out preexisting hypertension, nephropathy, and retinopathy at first booking, as described in pre-pregnancy planning.

Regular measurement of weight and blood pressure at each planned antenatal visit (every 1–2 weeks in early pregnancy, at least every 4 weeks in midpregnancy, and every week from 36 weeks gestation) is necessary to record gestational weight gain and early detection of hypertension and preeclampsia. Telephone or video telehealth consultations associated with home monitoring of glycemia and blood pressure may help reduce the burden of frequent clinic visits for some women. Patients with preexisting comorbid hypertension, nephropathy, and retinopathy need closer monitoring. There are no evidence-based protocols to guide the frequency and type of assessments, and these must be based on clinical judgment, local protocols, and resources. ADA recommends that all women must undergo dilated eye examination pre-pregnancy or at first booking, and in each trimester subsequently, and 1 year postpartum, as indicated by the degree of retinopathy and advised by the ophthalmologist.[71]

THERAPY TARGETS

The main goal of treatment is to ensure good metabolic control to prevent occurrence or progression of diabetes and pregnancy-related complications in the mother and

Table 1
Recommendations for glucose monitoring for pregnant women with type 2 DM

Recommendation for SMBG in Pregnancy with DM	Resource Setting	Strength of Recommendation and Quality of Evidence
SMBG is recommended for all pregnant women with diabetes, 3–4 times a day • Fasting: once daily, following at least 8 h of overnight fasting • Postprandial: 2–3 times daily, 1 or 2 h after the onset of meals, rotating meals on different days of the week	All	2|⊕ ⊕OO
SMBG is recommended for all pregnant women with diabetes at least once daily, with documented relation to timing of meal	Low	2|⊕OOO

survival, normal growth, and development of the fetus. The most important factors for attainment of this goal are normalization of glucose without undue hypoglycemia throughout pregnancy and during labor and delivery, preventing excess gestational weight gain, preventing preeclampsia, and treating comorbid hypertension.

Glucose control: optimal blood glucose levels for prevention of fetal risk have not been established. Data suggest that postprandial glucose levels more closely relate to macrosomia risk compared with fasting glucose levels.[80–82] Observational studies have shown correlation between glucose levels during labor and neonatal outcomes.[83,84] Maternal hyperglycemia during labor and delivery is associated with neonatal hypoglycemia, birth asphyxia, and nonreassuring fetal heart rate tracings.[85] **Table 2** provides recommendations based on ADA[71] and FIGO guidelines.[62]

Blood pressure control: in normal pregnancy blood pressure levels are lower owing to the generalized vasodilation. Pregnancy hypertension is defined as systolic blood pressure (BP) $\geq$140 mm Hg or diastolic BP $\geq$90 mm Hg. Tighter control of BP during pregnancy does not materially improve pregnancy outcome.[86] In pregnancies complicated by hypertension including those among women with diabetes blood pressure targets of 120 to 160/80 to 105 are considered reasonable.[87] Attempts to lower blood pressure below these levels are associated with impaired fetal growth.[71]

Gestational weight gain: weight reduction for obese and overweight women before pregnancy is advised. The Institute of Medicine (IOM) has published recommendations for weight gain during pregnancy, based on pre-pregnancy body mass index,[88] there is no recommendation specific to pregnancies complicated by diabetes. Some evidence suggests that weight reduction may be appropriate,[89] whereas other studies suggest that weight loss or $\leq$5 kg gain during pregnancy is associated with risk of small for gestational age deliveries.[90] IOM recommendations for weight gain during pregnancy are given in **Table 3**.

PRENATAL FOLLOW-UP

There is no evidence to support a particular protocol of antenatal follow-up for women with diabetes.[87] FIGO makes the following recommendation for prenatal follow-up in different resource settings (**Table 4**).[62]

Fetal sonographic assessment: because fetal macrosomia is the most frequent complication of diabetes, effort should be directed toward its diagnosis and prevention. Monitoring of fetal growth is both challenging and inaccurate with a $\pm$15% error margin. FIGO recommendation for the timing of sonographic assessments is shown in **Table 5**.[62]

Table 2
Recommendations for glycemic targets for diabetes in pregnancy

Glycemic Targets for Diabetes in Pregnancy[62,71]	Resource Setting	Strength of Recommendation and Quality of Evidence
Targets for glucose control during pregnancy • Fasting glucose <95 mg/dL (5.3 mmol/L) • 1 h postprandial <140 mg/dL (7.8 mmol/L) • 2 h postprandial <120 mg/dL (6.7 mmol/L)	All	1|⊕ ⊕OO
Target for glucose control during labor and delivery • 72–126 mg/dL (4–7 mmol/L)	All	1|⊕ ⊕ ⊕ ⊕

Table 3 IOM recommendations for weight gain during pregnancy		
Pre-pegnancy Body Mass Index (kg/m²)	Total Weight Gain (kg)	Rate of Weight Gain 2nd and 3rd Trimester Mean (Range) in kg/wk
Underweight, <18.5	12.5–18	0.51 (0.44–0.58)
Normal weight, 18.5–24.9	11.5–16	0.42 (0.35–0.50)
Overweight, 25.0–29.9	7–11.5	0.28 (0.23–0.33)
Obese, ≥30.0 kg/m²	5–9	0.22 (0.17–0.27)

Fetal Wellbeing

Fetal assessment can be achieved by a fetal kick count, biophysical profile, and non-stress test. There is no high quality evidence to suggest an optimal strategy for monitoring of fetal wellbeing. However, it is assumed that with reassuring fetal wellbeing, pregnancy prolongation to term can be achieved.[91]

Timing and mode of delivery: because of increased risk of intrauterine death and other adverse outcomes, induction of labor may be considered at 38 to 39 weeks, although there is no good-quality evidence to support such an approach. Some guidelines suggest that in pregnancies with good glycemic control and a seemingly appropriate estimated weight for gestational age, pregnancy ought to continue until 40 to 41 weeks.[87] Elective cesarean delivery may be considered when the best estimate of fetal weight exceeds 4000 g.[92,93] A decision flow chart for timing and mode of delivery in women with diabetes based on FIGO recommendation is shown in **Fig. 1.**

Nutritional therapy: medical nutritional therapy for diabetes is defined as: "a carbohydrate-controlled meal plan that promotes adequate nutrition with appropriate weight gain, normoglycemia and the absence of ketosis."[94] Nutrition intervention is the first line therapy in all pregnant women with diabetes,[71] and studies demonstrate that this results in improved metabolic control for type 2 DM.[95] Individualized meal plans should be culturally appropriate and based on eating habits, physical activity, blood glucose measurements, and physiologic effects of pregnancy.

Table 4 Recommendation for prenatal follow-up in different resource settings		
Recommendations for Prenatal Care for Women with DM[62]	Resource Setting	Strength of Recommendation and Quality of Evidence
Routine prenatal care should include visits to: • Perinatologist, diabetologist, diabetes educator: 1–3 wk as needed • Nurse—weight, blood pressure, dipstick urine protein: 1–2 wk as needed	High	1⏐⊕OOO
Prenatal care determined locally according to available resource: • At least monthly follow-up with a health care practitioner knowledgeable with diabetes • Refer to higher center if insulin treatment required or if comorbid conditions are present	Mid & Low	2⏐⊕OOO

Table 5
Recommendations for fetal growth assessment in DM

Recommendations for Fetal Growth Assessment in DM[62]	Resource Setting	Strength of Recommendation and Quality of Evidence
First trimester—ultrasonographic assessment for pregnancy dating and viability	High	1|⊕OOO
Second trimester—detailed anatomic ultrasonogram at 18–20 wk and a fetal echocardiogram if the blood sugars were elevated in the first trimester	High	1|⊕OOO
Clinical and sonographic growth assessments every 2–4 wk—starting at time of diagnosis until term	High	1|⊕OOO
Periodic clinical and sonographic growth assessments starting at time of diagnosis until term	Mid & Low	2|⊕OOO

Modest calorie restriction (1600–1800 calories/d, 33%) does not increase ketonuria and ketonemia.[96] Daily energy intake of approximately 2050 calories in all body mass index categories of women with diabetes is able to restrict undue gestational weight gain, maintain euglycemia, avoid ketonuria, and reduce risk of

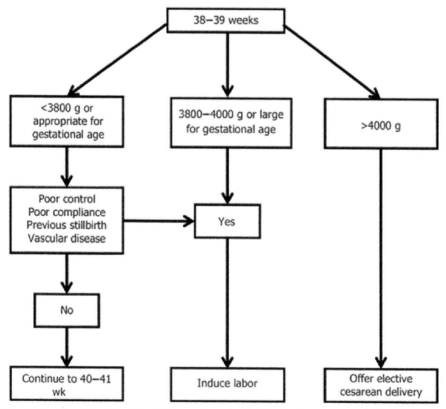

Fig. 1. Decision flow chart for timing and mode of delivery in women with diabetes.

macrosomia.[97] Focusing on the amount, quality, and distribution of carbohydrate can greatly help improve metabolic control in all patients with diabetes. A minimum of 175 g carbohydrates distributed throughout the day in 3 small- to moderate-sized meals and 2 to 4 snacks should be provided.[98] Low-glycemic-index foods help flatten prandial glucose spikes and reduce macrosomia risk, and are therefore considered the most appropriate dietary intervention in diabetes pregnancy.[99] Low glycemic index foods also have higher fiber content. Adequate fiber ingestion helps reduce constipation, a common problem in pregnancy. Up to 28 g fiber intake per day is recommended for women, and foods rich in fiber should be preferred. Pregnant women with diabetes must receive practical education that empowers them to choose the right quantity and quality of food. This can be achieved through teaching portion sizes, the plate model, and a culturally appropriate food pyramid or traffic sign concept. Nutritional education should highlight healthier cooking methods and how to reduce or moderate consumption of processed, high-sugar, high-fat, high-salt, and low-fiber foods.

Physical activity: physical activity in nonpregnant patients with diabetes improves metabolic control, reduces insulin resistance, cardiovascular risk, and improves weight control and overall wellbeing. Previously physically active women with type 2 DM without complications should be encouraged to continue pre-pregnancy physical activity levels with some moderation. Women should be advised to monitor fetal activity and blood glucose levels before and after exercise. Women with past bad obstetric histories, or with complications, must be individually assessed and counseled regarding permissible physical activities.

PHARMACOLOGIC TREATMENT OF TYPE 2 DIABETES IN PREGNANCY

Insulin is the preferred agent for treatment of type 2 DM in pregnancy because it does not cross the placenta, and because oral agents are generally insufficient to overcome the insulin resistance in type 2 DM.[71] Pregnant women should ideally receive basal/bolus insulin treatment; in which <50% of the total daily dose should be given as basal insulin and greater than 50% as prandial insulin matched to meal time and size. In the first trimester, insulin-treated women with type 2 DM, just like women with type 1 DM, may experience a decrease in insulin requirements. In the second trimester, rapidly increasing insulin resistance will require weekly or biweekly insulin dose titration to maintain glycemic targets. Late in the third trimester, there may be a leveling off of, or a small decrease in, insulin requirement. The physiology of pregnancy necessitates frequent dose titration and underlines the importance of SMBG and team-based care when resources are available.

Although glycemic control maybe easier to achieve in pregnant women with type 2 DM than with type 1 DM, relative insulin requirements are much higher throughout pregnancy and drop dramatically after delivery. Insulin sensitivity increases with delivery of the placenta and returns to pre-pregnancy levels over the following 1 to 2 weeks. Many women with type 2 DM may be able to cease insulin treatment in the immediate postnatal period. In women taking insulin, particular attention should be directed to hypoglycemia prevention in the setting of breastfeeding and erratic sleep and eating schedules.

The use of oral drugs to treat type 2 DM in pregnancy remains contentious because these drugs cross the placental barrier and lack adequate long-term safety data. Oral drugs, particularly metformin and glyburide, are being increasingly accepted and used to treat women with gestational diabetes,[62] with less concern for short-term untoward effects and safety, particularly when used later during pregnancy. Other than metformin and glyburide, no other oral drug has data to merit consideration for use during pregnancy. Long-term effects on offspring remain unclear, but, based on limited data, raise no alarms as yet when used in women with GDM.[100] Their use in women with pre-pregnancy type 2 DM and DIP during the early stages of pregnancy, particularly during the period of organogenesis, raises concern both from the toxicity perspective (due to placental transfer), and limited ability and flexibility to control blood sugar compared with insulin during critical developmental phases.

Sulfonylurea derivatives are typically recommended for patients with 2 of the most frequent forms of transcription factor-linked MODY: HNF1-α and HNF4-α. During pregnancy in these cases use of glyburide is justified. Use of nonsulfonylurea secretagogs (glinides), with lower incidence of hypoglycemia, may also be considered but their safety in pregnancy is even less known.[101]

Metformin use in pregnant women with type 2 DM has been assessed in a few observational and small randomized trials.[102–104] Metformin monotherapy in pregnant women with overt diabetes may fail to achieve glycemic targets, but its use as an adjunct to insulin in women with high insulin requirements or those showing rapid weight gain may be considered. There is a need for more trials to assess the effect of combined (insulin plus metformin) therapy in pregnancy with type 2 DM. The results of the ongoing metformin in women with type 2 DM in pregnancy (MiTy) trial,[105] when available, will inform and likely impact the management of pregnant women with type 2 DM.

In women refusing insulin treatment, or in situations in which insulin therapy is not available or cannot be safely administered and monitored, there may be no option but to use metformin or glyburide.

Management of hypertension and nephropathy in DIP: as well as strict glycemic control before and during pregnancy, early and intensive antihypertensive treatment is important to optimize pregnancy outcomes. Methyldopa, labetalol, nifedipine, and diltiazem are considered safe, whereas ACE inhibitors or angiotensin receptor blockers should be stopped before or at confirmation of pregnancy. Supplementation with folic acid in early pregnancy and low-dose aspirin from 10 to 12 weeks reduces the risk of preeclampsia-related adverse outcomes.

Prevention of preeclampsia: the American College of Obstetricians and Gynecologists, the US Preventive Services Task Force,[106] and the ADA[71] recommend that low-dose aspirin prophylaxis at 81 mg/d from 12 and 28 weeks' gestation (optimally at <16 weeks' gestation), continued daily until delivery, should be given to pregnant women with type 2 DM. The currently published Aspirin for Evidence-Based Preeclampsia Prevention (ASPRE) trial shows that the rate of delivery with preterm preeclampsia (preterm PE) can be reduced by 62% by aspirin started at 11 to 14 weeks' gestation in high-risk women.[107] The ASPRE trial used a combination of risk factors and screening tests including biomarkers to identify women at risk, and was designed to test the hypothesis that aspirin at a dose of 150 mg per night from 11 to 14 until 36 weeks' gestation, compared with placebo, would result in halving the incidence of preterm PE. Results from the ASPRE trial are definitive proof that effective screening for preterm PE can be achieved with combined test of maternal factors and biomarkers at 11 to 13 weeks, and that high-risk women can take aspirin 150 mg per night from the first trimester of pregnancy to significantly reduce their chances of developing preterm PE. Administration of aspirin was safe and reduced the length of stay in the NICU by about 68%. The findings have implications for short-term and long-term health care costs and savings as well as infant survival, disability, and human capital.

IMMEDIATE AND LONG-TERM POSTPARTUM MANAGEMENT

Being vulnerable to multiple complications women with type 2 DM and their offspring need careful monitoring immediately after delivery. Further discussion on it is beyond the scope of this review. Suffice it to say that pregnancy is a major event in any woman's life, and in the postpartum period the focus tends to shift from the mother's health to the nurturing of the baby. However, for a woman with type 2 DM, postpartum care and follow-up are vital to ensuring immediate and long-term health for herself, her child, and their family.

Promotion of breast feeding is an essential element of postnatal care and has been shown to reduce longer term risk of diabetes in the offspring,[108] although specific data for mothers with type 2 DM are lacking. It is important to maintain an active focus on the mothers' health, despite the obvious pressing needs of the baby, both in the immediate postnatal period and in the longer term. Cardiovascular disease is the major long-term threat to the health of women with type 2 DM[109] and active postpartum management is essential, aimed at improving lifestyle factors through modification of diet and physical activity patterns and managing hyperglycemia and other important cardiovascular risk factors such as hypertension, hyperlipidemia, and smoking cessation.

REFERENCES

1. International diabetes federation IDF diabetes atlas 7th Edition. Available at: http://www.diabetesatlas.org/. Accessed October 15, 2018.
2. World Health Organization. Obesity and overweight fact sheet Updated June 2016. Available at: http://www.who.int/mediacentre/factsheets/fs311/en/. Accessed October 15, 2018.
3. Albrecht SS, Kuklina EV, Bansil P, et al. Diabetes trends among delivery hospitalizations in the U.S., 1994-2004. Diabetes Care 2010;33(4):768–73.
4. Bardenheier BH, Imperatore G, Devlin HM, et al. Trends in pre-pregnancy diabetes among deliveries in 19 U.S. states, 2000-2010. Am J Prev Med 2015; 48(2):154–61.
5. Mackin ST, Nelson SM, Kerssens JJ, et al. SDRN epidemiology group diabetes and pregnancy: national trends over a 15 year period. Diabetologia 2018;61(5): 1081–8.
6. Bell R, Bailey K, Cresswell T, et al. Trends in prevalence and outcomes of pregnancy in women with pre-existing type I and type II diabetes. BJOG 2008;115: 445–52.
7. Fadl HE, Simmons D. Trends in diabetes in pregnancy in Sweden 1998-2012. BMJ Open Diabetes Res Care 2016;4(1):e000221.
8. Metcalfe A, Sabr Y, Hutcheon JA, et al. Trends in obstetric intervention and pregnancy outcomes of canadian women with diabetes in pregnancy from 2004 to 2015. J Endocr Soc 2017;1(12):1540–9.
9. Zhou Q, Wang Q, Shen H, et al. Prevalence of diabetes and regional differences in Chinese women planning pregnancy: a nationwide population-based cross-sectional study. Diabetes Care 2017;40:e16–8.
10. Kragelund Nielsen K, Damm P, Kapur A, et al. Risk factors for hyperglycaemia in pregnancy in Tamil Nadu, India. PLoS One 2016;11(3):e0151311.
11. World Health Organization. Diagnostic criteria and classification of hyperglycaemia first detected in pregnancy. WHO/NMH/MND/13.2; 2013. Available at: https://apps.who.int/iris/bitstream/handle/10665/85975/WHO_NMH_MND_13.2_

eng.pdf;jsessionid=7680B9F80A5977C8F21A26419BBFEB3F?sequence=1. Accessed October 15, 2018.

12. Shields BM, Hicks S, Shepherd MH, et al. Maturity-onset diabetes of the young (MODY): how many cases are we missing? Diabetologia 2010;53:2504–8.

13. Kropff J, Selwood MP, McCarthy MI, et al. Prevalence of monogenic diabetes in young adults: a community-based, cross-sectional study in Oxfordshire, UK. Diabetologia 2011;54:1261–3.

14. Pihoker C, Gilliam LK, Ellard S, et al. Prevalence, characteristics and clinical diagnosis of maturity onset diabetes of the young due to mutations in HNF1A, HNF4A, and glucokinase: results from the SEARCH for Diabetes in Youth. J Clin Endocrinol Metab 2013;98:4055–62.

15. OMIM - Online Mendelian Inheritance in man. 2016. Available at: http://www.omim.org/.

16. Ellard S, Beards F, Allen L, et al. A high prevalence of glucokinase mutations in gestational diabetic subjects selected by clinical criteria. Diabetologia 2000; 43(2):250–3.

17. Doddabelavangala MM, Chapla A, Hesarghatta Shyamasunder A, et al. Comprehensive maturity onset diabetes of the young (MODY) gene screening in pregnant women with diabetes in India. PLoS One 2017;12(1):e0168656.

18. Angueira AR, Ludvik AE, Reddy TE, et al. New insights into gestational glucose metabolism: lessons learned from 21st century approaches. Diabetes 2015;64: 327–34.

19. Dekel N, Gnainsky Y, Granot I, et al. Inflammation and implantation. Am J Reprod Immunol 2010;63:17–21.

20. Mor G, Cardenas I. The immune system in pregnancy: a unique complexity. Am J Reprod Immunol 2010;63:425–33.

21. Romero R, Espinoza J, Goncalves LF, et al. Inflammation in preterm and term labor and delivery. Semin Fetal Neonatal Med 2006;11:317–26.

22. Newbern D, Freemark M. Placental hormones and the control of maternal metabolism and fetal growth. Curr Opin Endocrinol Diabetes Obes 2011;18:409–16.

23. Butler AE, Cao-Minh L, Galasso R, et al. Adaptive changes in pancreatic beta cell fractional area and beta cell turnover in human pregnancy. Diabetologia 2010;53:2167–76.

24. Jacovetti C, Abderrahmani A, Parnaud G, et al. MicroRNAs contribute to compensatory B cell expansion during pregnancy and obesity. J Clin Invest 2012;122:3541–51.

25. Catalano PM. Trying to understand gestational diabetes. Diabet Med 2014;31: 273–81.

26. Wang M, Xia W, Li H, et al. Normal pregnancy induced glucose metabolic stress in a longitudinal cohort of healthy women: novel insights generated from a urine metabolomics study. Medicine (Baltimore) 2018;97:e12417.

27. Baeyens L, Hindi S, Sorenson RL, et al. Beta-cell adaptation in pregnancy. Diabetes Obes Metab 2016;18(Suppl 1):63–70.

28. Nelson SM, Matthews P, Poston L. Maternal metabolism and obesity: modifiable determinants of pregnancy outcome. Hum Reprod Update 2010;16(3):255–75.

29. Desoye G, Nolan CJ. The fetal glucose steal: an underappreciated phenomenon in diabetic pregnancy. Diabetologia 2016;59(6):1089–94.

30. Metzger BE, Lowe LP, Dyer AR, et al. Hyperglycemia and adverse pregnancy outcomes. N Engl J Med 2008;358:1991–2002.

31. Freinkel N. Banting lecture 1980. Of pregnancy and progeny. Diabetes 1980;29: 1023–35.

32. Carpenter MW, Canick JA, Hogan JW, et al. Amniotic fluid insulin at 14-20 weeks gestation: association with later maternal glucose intolerance and birth macrosomia. Diabetes care 2001;24:1259–63.
33. Schwartz R, Gruppuso PA, Petzold K, et al. Hyperinsulinemia and macrosomia in the fetus of the diabetic mother. Diabetes Care 1994;17:640–8.
34. Starikov R, Inman K, Chen K, et al. Comparison of placental findings in type 1 and type 2 diabetic pregnancies. Placenta 2014;35:1001–6.
35. Gabbay-Benziv R, Baschat AA. Gestational diabetes as one of the "great obstetrical syndromes"—the maternal, placental, and fetal dialog. Best Pract Res Clin Obstet Gynaecol 2015;29:150–5.
36. Balsells M, García-Patterson A, Gich I, et al. Maternal and fetal outcome in women with type 2 versus type 1 diabetes mellitus: a systematic review and metaanalysis. J Clin Endocrinol Metab 2009;94:4284–91.
37. Billionnet C, Mitanchez D, Weill A, et al. Gestational diabetes and adverse perinatal outcomes from 716,152 births in France in 2012. Diabetologia 2017;60: 636–44.
38. Wahabi H, Fayed A, Esmaeil S, et al. Prevalence and complications of pregestational and gestational diabetes in Saudi women: analysis from Riyadh mother and baby cohort study (RAHMA). Biomed Res Int 2017;2017:6878263.
39. Nielsen GL, Nogard B, Puho E, et al. Risk of specific congenital abnormalities in offspring of women with diabetes. Diabet Med 2005;22:693–6.
40. Dart AB, Ruth CA, Sellers EA, et al. Maternal diabetes mellitus and congenital anomalies of the kidney and urinary tract (CAKUT) in the child. Am J Kidney Dis 2015;65:684–91.
41. Liu S, Rouleau J, León JA, Canadian Perinatal Surveillance System, et al. Impact of pre-pregnancy diabetes mellitus on congenital anomalies, Canada, 2002-2012. Health Promot Chronic Dis Prev Can 2015;35:79–84.
42. Jovanovič L, Liang Y, Weng W, et al. Trends in the incidence of diabetes, its clinical sequelae, and associated costs in pregnancy. Diabetes Metab Res Rev 2015;31:707–16.
43. Serehi AA, Ahmed AM, Shakeel F, et al. A comparison on the prevalence and outcomes of gestational versus type 2 diabetes mellitus in 1718 Saudi pregnancies. Int J Clin Exp Med 2015;8:11502–7.
44. Klingensmith GJ, Pyle L, Nadeau KJ, TODAY Study Group, et al. Pregnancy outcomes in youth with type 2 diabetes: the TODAY study experience. Diabetes Care 2016;39(1):122–9.
45. Wicklow BA, Sellers EAC, Sharma AK, et al. Association of gestational diabetes and type 2 diabetes exposure in utero with the development of type 2 diabetes in first nations and non-first nations offspring. JAMA Pediatr 2018;172(8): 724–31.
46. Clausen TD, Mathiesen ER, Hansen T, et al. High prevalence of type 2 diabetes and pre-diabetes in adult offspring of women with gestational diabetes mellitus or type 1 diabetes: the role of intrauterine hyperglycemia. Diabetes Care 2008; 31(2):340–6.
47. Dabelea D, Mayer-Davis EJ, Lamichhane AP, et al. Association of intrauterine exposure to maternal diabetes and obesity with type 2 diabetes in youth: the SEARCH Case-Control Study. Diabetes Care 2008;31:1422–6.
48. Pettitt DJ, Lawrence JM, Beyer J, et al. Association between maternal diabetes in utero and age at offspring's diagnosis of type 2 diabetes. Diabetes Care 2008;31:2126–30.

49. Ornoy A. Growth and neurodevelopmental outcome of children born to mothers with pregestational and gestational diabetes. Pediatr Endocrinol Rev 2005;3: 104–13.

50. Xiang AH, Wang X, Martinez MP, et al. Maternal gestational diabetes mellitus, type 1 diabetes, and type 2 diabetes during pregnancy and risk of ADHD in offspring. Diabetes Care 2018. https://doi.org/10.2337/dc18-0733.

51. Li M, Fallin MD, Riley A, et al. The association of maternal obesity and diabetes with autism and other developmental disabilities. Pediatrics 2016;137(2): e20152206.

52. Xu G, Jing J, Bowers K, et al. Maternal diabetes and the risk of autism spectrum disorders in the offspring: a systematic review and meta-analysis. J Autism Dev Disord 2014;44:766–75.

53. Rasmussen KL, Laugesen CS, Ringholm L, et al. Progression of diabetic retinopathy during pregnancy in women with type 2 diabetes. Diabetologia 2010; 53:1076–83.

54. Egan AM, McVicker L, Heerey A, et al. Diabetic retinopathy in pregnancy: a population-based study of women with pre-gestational diabetes. J Diabetes Res 2015;2015:310239.

55. Makwana T, Takkar B, Venkatesh P, et al. Prevalence, progression, and outcomes of diabetic retinopathy during pregnancy in Indian scenario. Indian J Ophthalmol 2018;66:541–6.

56. Kitzmiller JL, Block JM, Brown FM, et al. Managing preexisting diabetes for pregnancy: summary of evidence and consensus recommendations for care. Diabetes Care 2008;31:1060–79.

57. Eppens MC, Craig ME, Jones TW, et al. International Diabetes Federation Western Pacific Region Steering Committee. Type 2 diabetes in youth from the Western Pacific region: glycaemic control, diabetes care and complications. Curr Med Res Opin 2006;22:1013–20.

58. Damm JA, Asbjörnsdóttir B, Callesen NF, et al. Diabetic nephropathy and microalbuminuria in pregnant women with type 1 and type 2 diabetes: prevalence, antihypertensive strategy, and pregnancy outcome. Diabetes Care 2013;36: 3489–94.

59. Dart AB, Sellers EA, Martens PJ, et al. High burden of kidney disease in youth-onset type 2 diabetes. Diabetes Care 2012;35:1265–71.

60. Bramham K. Diabetic nephropathy and pregnancy. Semin Nephrol 2017;37: 362–9.

61. Ringholm L, Damm JA, Vestgaard M, et al. Diabetic nephropathy in women with preexisting diabetes: from pregnancy planning to breastfeeding. Curr Diab Rep 2016;16:12.

62. Hod M, Kapur A, Sacks DA, et al. The International Federation of Gynecology and Obstetrics (FIGO) Initiative on gestational diabetes mellitus: a pragmatic guide for diagnosis, management, and care. Int J Gynaecol Obstet 2015; 131(Suppl 3):S173–211.

63. Cea-Soriano L, García-Rodríguez LA, Brodovicz KG, et al. Real world management of pregestational diabetes not achieving glycemic control for many patients in the UK. Pharmacoepidemiol Drug Saf 2018;27(8):940–8.

64. Sina M, MacMillan F, Dune T, et al. Development of an integrated, district-wide approach to pre-pregnancy management for women with pre-existing diabetes in a multi-ethnic population. BMC Pregnancy Childbirth 2018;18:402.

65. Klein J, Boyle JA, Kirkham R, et al. Preconception care for women with type 2 diabetes mellitus: a mixed-methods study of provider knowledge and practice. Diabetes Res Clin Pract 2017;129:105–15.
66. Murphy HR, Bell R, Dornhorst A, et al. Pregnancy in diabetes: challenges and opportunities for improving pregnancy outcomes. Diabet Med 2018;35:292–9.
67. Yamamoto JM, Hughes DJF, Evans ML, et al. Community-based pre-pregnancy care programme improves pregnancy preparation in women with pregestational diabetes. Diabetologia 2018. https://doi.org/10.1007/s00125-018-4613-3.
68. Owens LA, Egan AM, Carmody L, et al. Ten years of optimizing outcomes for women with type 1 and type 2 diabetes in pregnancy - the Atlantic DIP experience. J Clin Endocrinol Metab 2016;101:1598–605.
69. Egan AM, Danyliv A, Carmody L, et al. A pre pregnancy care program for women with diabetes: effective and cost saving. J Clin Endocrinol Metab 2016;101:1807–15.
70. Peterson C, Grosse SD, Li R, et al. Preventable health and cost burden of adverse birth outcomes associated with pregestational diabetes in the United States. Am J Obstet Gynecol 2015;212:74.e1-9.
71. American Diabetes Association. Management of diabetes in pregnancy: standards of medical care in diabetes-2018. Diabetes Care 2018;41(Suppl 1): S137–43.
72. Gourdy P. Diabetes and oral contraception. Best Pract Res Clin Endocrinol Metab 2013;27(1):67–76. https://doi.org/10.1016/j.beem.2012.11.001.
73. Parks C, Peipert JF. Eliminating health disparities in unintended pregnancy with long-acting reversible contraception (LARC). Am J Obstet Gynecol 2016;214: 681–8.
74. Jovanovic LG. Using meal-based self-monitoring of blood glucose as a tool to improve outcomes in pregnancy complicated by diabetes. Endocr Pract 2008;14:239–47.
75. Moy FM, Ray A, Buckley BS, et al. Techniques of monitoring blood glucose during pregnancy for women with pre-existing diabetes. Cochrane Database Syst Rev 2017;(6):CD009613.
76. Murphy HR, Rayman G, Lewis K, et al. Effectiveness of continuous glucose monitoring in pregnant women with diabetes: randomised clinical trial. BMJ 2008;337:a1680.
77. Secher AL, Ringholm L, Andersen HU, et al. The effect of real-time continuous glucose monitoring in pregnant women with diabetes: a randomized controlled trial. Diabetes care 2013;36:1877–83.
78. Voormolen DN, DeVries JH, Sanson RME, et al. Continuous glucose monitoring during diabetic pregnancy (GlucoMOMS): a multicentre randomized controlled trial. Diabetes Obes Metab 2018;20:1894–902.
79. Feig DS, Donovan LE, Corcoy R, CONCEPTT Collaborative Group, et al. Continuous glucose monitoring in pregnant women with type 1 diabetes (CONCEPTT): a multicenter international randomised controlled trial. Lancet 2017;390(10110): 2347–59 [Erratum in: Lancet 2017;390(10110):2346].
80. deVeciana M, Major CA, Morgan MA. Postprandial versus preprandial blood glucose monitoring in women with gestational diabetes mellitus requiring insulin therapy. N Engl J Med 1995;333:1237–41.
81. Combs CA, Gunderson E, Kitsmiller JL. Relationship of fetal macrosomia to maternal postprandial glucose control during pregnancy. Diabetes Care 1992; 15:1251–7.

82. Jovanovic L, Peterson CM, Reed GF. Maternal postprandial glucose levels and infant birth weight: the Diabetes in Early Pregnancy study. Am J Obstet Gynecol 1991;164:103–11.

83. Andersen O, Hertel J, Schmølker L, et al. Influence of the maternal plasma glucose concentration at delivery on the risk of hypoglycaemia in infants of insulin-dependent diabetic mothers. Acta Paediatr Scand 1985;74(2):268–73.

84. Curet LB, Izquierdo LA, Gilson GJ, et al. Relative effects of antepartum and intrapartum maternal blood glucose levels on incidence of neonatal hypoglycemia. J Perinatol 1997;17(2):113–5.

85. Mimouni F, Miodovnik M, Siddiqi TA, et al. Perinatal asphyxia in infants of insulin-dependent diabetic mothers. J Pediatr 1988;113(2):345–53.

86. Magee LA, von Dadelszen P, Rey E, et al. Less-tight versus tight control of hypertension in pregnancy. N Engl J Med 2015;372(5):407–17.

87. American College of Obstetricians and Gynecologists; Task Force on Hypertension in Pregnancy. Hypertension in pregnancy. Report of the American College of Obstetricians and Gynecologists' Task Force on Hypertension in Pregnancy. Obstet Gynecol 2013;122(5):1122–31.

88. Institute of Medicine. Weight gain during pregnancy: reexamining the guidelines. Washington, DC: National Academies Press (US); 2009.

89. Artal R, Catanzaro RB, Gavard JA, et al. A lifestyle intervention of weight-gain restriction: diet and exercise in obese women with gestational diabetes mellitus. Appl Physiol Nutr Metab 2007;32(3):596–601.

90. Catalano PM, Mele L, Landon MB, et al. Inadequate weight gain in overweight and obese pregnant women: what is the effect on fetal growth? Am J Obstet Gynecol 2014;211(2):137.e1–7.

91. Committee on Practice Bulletins–Obstetrics. Practice Bulletin No. 137: Gestational diabetes mellitus. Obstet Gynecol 2013;122(2 Pt 1):406–16.

92. Yogev Y, Ben-Haroush A, Chen R, et al. Active induction management of labor for diabetic pregnancies at term; mode of delivery and fetal outcome–a single center experience. Eur J Obstet Gynecol Reprod Biol 2004;114(2):166–70.

93. American College of Obstetricians and Gynecologists (College); Society for Maternal-Fetal Medicine, Caughey AB, Cahill AG, Guise JM, et al. Safe prevention of the primary cesarean delivery. Am J Obstet Gynecol 2014;210(3):179–93.

94. American Dietetic Association, Medical Nutrition Therapy Evidence Based Guide for Practice: Nutrition Practice Guidelines for Gestational Diabetes [CD.ROM]. Chicago (IL): American Dietetic Association; 2001.

95. Franz MJ, Monk A, Barry B, et al. Effectiveness of medical nutrition therapy provided by dietitians in the management of non-insulin-dependent diabetes mellitus: a randomized, controlled clinical trial. J Am Diet Assoc 1995;95:1009–17.

96. American Diabetes Association. Gestational diabetes mellitus. Diabetes Care 2004;27(Suppl 1):S88–90.

97. Snyder J, Gray-Donald K, Koski KG. Predictors of infant birth weight in gestational diabetes. Am J Clin Nutr 1994;59(6):1409–14.

98. Institute of Medicine. Dietary reference intakes: energy, carbohydrate, fiber, fat, fatty acids, cholesterol, protein, and amino acids. Washington, DC: National Academies Press; 2002.

99. Viana LV, Gross JL, Azevedo MJ. Dietary intervention in patients with gestational diabetes mellitus: a systematic review and meta-analysis of randomized clinical trials on maternal and newborn outcomes. Diabetes Care 2014;37(12):3345–55.

100. Ekpebegh CO, Coetzee EJ, van derMerwe L, et al. A 10-year retrospective analysis of pregnancy outcome in pregestational type 2 diabetes: comparison of insulin and oral glucose-lowering agents. Diabet Med 2007;24:253–8.
101. Brunerova L, Rahelić D, Ceriello A, et al. Use of oral antidiabetic drugs in the treatment of maturity-onset diabetes of the young: a mini review. Diabetes Metab Res Rev 2018;34(1). https://doi.org/10.1002/dmrr.2940.
102. Hickman MA, McBride R, Boggess KA, et al. Metformin compared with insulin in the treatment of pregnant women with overt diabetes: a randomized controlled trial. Am J Perinatol 2013;30(6):483–90.
103. Ainuddin JA, Karim N, Zaheer S, et al. Metformin treatment in type 2 diabetes in pregnancy: an active controlled, parallel-group, randomized, open label study in patients with type 2 diabetes in pregnancy. J Diabetes Res 2015;2015: 325851.
104. Gilbert C, Valois M, Koren G. Pregnancy outcome after first-trimester exposure to metformin: a meta-analysis. Fertil Steril 2006;86(3):658–63.
105. Feig DS, Murphy K, Asztalos E, on behalf of the MiTy Collabortive Group, et al. Metformin in women with type 2 diabetes in pregnancy (MiTy): a multi-center randomized controlled trial. BMC Pregnancy Childbirth 2016;16(1):173.
106. Henderson JT, Whitlock EP, O'Connor E, et al. Low-dose aspirin for prevention of morbidity and mortality from preeclampsia: a systematic evidence review for the U.S Preventive Services Task Force. Annals of Internal Medicine 2014;160(10): 695–703.
107. Rolnik DL, Wright D, Poon LC, et al. Aspirin versus placebo in pregnancies at high risk for preterm preeclampsia. N Engl J Med 2017;377(7):613–22.
108. Horta BL, Loret de Mola C, Victora CG. Long-term consequences of breastfeeding on cholesterol, obesity, systolic blood pressure and type 2 diabetes: a systematic review and meta-analysis. Acta Paediatr 2015;104(467):30–7.
109. Retnakaran R. Hyperglycemia in pregnancy and its implications for a woman's future risk of cardiovascular disease. Diabetes Res Clin Pract 2018. https://doi.org/10.1016/j.diabres.2018.04.008.

Hyperthyroidism and Pregnancy

Kristen Kobaly, MD*, Susan J. Mandel, MD, MPH

KEYWORDS

- Hyperthyroidism • Gestational thyrotoxicosis • Graves' disease • Lactation
- Thionamides • Teratogenicity • TRAb

KEY POINTS

- Appropriate diagnosis and treatment of thyrotoxicosis in pregnancy is necessary to prevent poor maternal and fetal outcomes, including pregnancy loss.
- Human chorionic gonadotropin–mediated gestational thyrotoxicosis, often associated with hyperemesis gravidarum, is a self-limited condition affecting 1% to 3% of pregnancies. Antithyroid drugs are not indicated for this condition.
- Graves' disease, the most common cause of clinically significant hyperthyroidism in pregnancy, may flare at around 10 to 15 weeks gestation and remit in later pregnancy, but often relapses postpartum.
- Because of teratogenicity, the lowest possible dose of antithyroid drug should be used to treat Graves' disease in pregnancy, with consideration of discontinuing the drug in early pregnancy.
- In women with a current or prior history of Graves' disease, pregnancies at risk for fetal/neonatal hyperthyroidism should be identified via serum thyrotropin receptor antibody measurements.

DIFFERENTIAL DIAGNOSIS AND EPIDEMIOLOGY OF HYPERTHYROIDISM IN PREGNANCY

Clinical thyrotoxicosis complicates 0.1% to 0.4% of pregnancies.[1] Although the differential diagnosis of thyrotoxicosis in pregnancy includes any cause that can be seen in a nonpregnant patient, the most likely causes are gestational thyrotoxicosis with or without hyperemesis gravidarum or Graves' disease. Gestational thyrotoxicosis is diagnosed in 1% to 3% of pregnancies, although two-thirds of patients with hyperemesis gravidarum are biochemically hyperthyroid.[2,3] Between ages 30 to 40 years, 0.5%

Disclosure: The authors have nothing to disclose.
Division of Endocrinology, Diabetes and Metabolism, Perelman School of Medicine, University of Pennsylvania, Perelman Center for Advanced Medicine, 4th Floor West Pavilion, 3400 Civic Center Boulevard, Philadelphia, PA 19104, USA
* Corresponding author.
E-mail address: Kristen.Kobaly@uphs.upenn.edu

Endocrinol Metab Clin N Am 48 (2019) 533–545
https://doi.org/10.1016/j.ecl.2019.05.002
0889-8529/19/© 2019 Elsevier Inc. All rights reserved.

endo.theclinics.com

to 1.3% of women who become pregnant have previously diagnosed Graves' disease; the theoretic risk of new-onset Graves' disease in pregnancy is about 0.05%.[4] Post-partum thyroiditis can occur up to a year from a prior pregnancy and may occur in pregnant women with an antecedent miscarriage or a short interpregnancy interval. Functional thyroid nodules are rare in women of childbearing age and are more common in iodine-insufficient regions. Rarer causes of hyperthyroidism are beyond the scope of this article.

Although no adverse pregnancy outcomes have been reported with subclinical hyperthyroidism,[5] overt hyperthyroidism and thyroid storm are associated with poor fetal and maternal obstetric outcomes. A 28-year retrospective study of pregnancies complicated by controlled or uncontrolled hyperthyroidism compared with age-matched and parity-matched controls found intrauterine growth restriction, placental abruption, preterm labor/birth, low birth weight, and stillbirth were increased in uncontrolled hyperthyroidism.[6] Severe preeclampsia and heart failure may also occur,[7,8] and thyroid storm has been reported. Therefore, appropriately differentiating and treating these conditions during pregnancy is important for maternal and fetal well-being.

GESTATIONAL THYROTOXICOSIS
Pathophysiology

Human chorionic gonadotropin (hCG) is a heterodimeric glycoprotein produced by the corpus luteum and the placenta. Levels of hCG increase rapidly in early pregnancy and peak around 10 weeks gestation, following which they subsequently decline until the third trimester and then remain stable for the duration of the pregnancy. The beta subunit of hCG shares structural homology with thyroid stimulating hormone (TSH); therefore, hCG can weakly stimulate the TSH receptor, increasing thyroidal hormone production and contributing to the lower TSH level observed at the end of the first trimester. A study that assessed thyroid function in more than 300 pregnant women found that 18% had transient low TSH ($\leq$0.20 mU/L) in the first trimester; in nearly 50% TSH was completely suppressed (<0.05 mU/L). Increased free thyroxine (T4) levels were seen in 10% of the suppressed TSH group, typically in association with vomiting.[9] In hyperemesis gravidarum, a condition that may be correlated with higher hCG levels, overt biochemical hyperthyroidism (suppressed TSH, increased free T4) is seen in two-thirds of patients, often in the absence of clinical symptoms of thyrotoxicosis, and resolves with resolution of the hyperemesis.[2,3] The severity of hyperemesis correlates with the magnitude of thyroid dysfunction.[10] Twin pregnancies are associated with higher and more prolonged hCG increase than singleton pregnancies and hence may have more profound TSH suppression with free T4 increase.[11]

Diagnosis

Signs and symptoms of hyperthyroidism in pregnancy (heat intolerance, increased heart rate, dyspnea, and wide pulse pressure) overlap considerably with normal physiologic changes of pregnancy, making diagnosis challenging. Clinical features that suggest a diagnosis of Graves' disease include goiter, which may appear hypervascular on ultrasonography[12]; tachycardia with a pulse more than 120 beats/min[3]; and ophthalmopathy. Weight loss occurs in both hyperemesis gravidarum and Graves' disease and does not differentiate these conditions.[3] Thyrotropin (TSH) receptor antibodies (TRAb) should be measured in suspected Graves' disease cases to confirm the diagnosis. Increased triiodothyronine (T3) levels and a high T3/T4 ratio also suggest Graves' disease.[13] Thyroid scintigraphy is contraindicated in pregnancy because of concerns for fetal radiation exposure.

Thyroid function tests in gestational thyrotoxicosis typically normalize within 10 weeks from diagnosis.[2] A study of gestational thyrotoxicosis associated with hyperemesis gravidarum found free T4 levels typically normalized by 15 weeks, whereas TSH remained suppressed through 19 weeks.[3] Persistent hyperthyroidism beyond these time points requires evaluation for an alternate diagnosis.

Management

Women with gestational thyrotoxicosis generally require no treatment. Antithyroid drugs (ATDs) are not recommended because of the transient nature of the abnormalities, risk of maternal/fetal hypothyroidism, and concern for teratogenicity. Thyroid function tests should be followed periodically through resolution of the abnormalities with monitoring for a hypothyroid phase if there is suspicion for transient autoimmune thyroiditis as an alternate diagnosis. β-Blockers may be considered; details of the use of these drugs in pregnancy is discussed further later. Hyperemesis gravidarum requires supportive care, including antiemetics, intravenous fluids, and correction of electrolytes abnormalities, if severe.

GRAVES' DISEASE IN PREGNANCY

Graves' disease may present for the first time during pregnancy or postpartum. A recent population-based cohort study using the Danish nationwide registry found the incidence ratio of hyperthyroidism to be high in the first 3 months of pregnancy, very low in the last 3 months, and highest at 7 to 9 months postpartum.[14] For women with known Graves' disease, exacerbation or relapse may occur by 10 to 15 weeks gestation.[15] In the late second or third trimester, a period of immune tolerance, patients often enter remission,[15] a process that correlates with decreases in TRAb levels.[16,17] Disease may relapse postpartum as TRAb levels increase,[15–17] with the greatest risk occurring around 7 to 9 months following delivery.[14,15,18] There is a 2-fold to 4-fold increased risk of new-onset Graves' disease in the postpartum period.[14]

PRECONCEPTION THERAPY FOR WOMEN WITH PREEXISTING GRAVES' DISEASE

In women with Graves' disease interested in childbearing, therapeutic considerations include the time course of planned conception, disease history and activity, and TRAb levels. A discussion of the risk of birth defects from ATDs should occur. If ATDs are continued, women may either be treated with propylthiouracil (PTU) before conceiving or changed to PTU as soon a pregnancy is confirmed.[19,20] Definitive treatment is often preferable unless disease course is mild or pregnancy is imminent. Hyperthyroidism should be controlled for several months before attempting pregnancy, and, if radioactive iodine or surgery are used, hypothyroidism should be treated with levothyroxine to achieve a euthyroid state before trying to conceive. Pregnancy should be avoided for 6 months following radioactive iodine.

Management

Treatment of Graves' disease in pregnancy must balance control of maternal hyperthyroidism while maintaining a euthyroid state in the fetus and avoiding adverse fetal side effects from therapeutic agents. Both ATDs and TRAb cross the placenta, affecting maternal and fetal thyroid status, and fetal screening for hyperthyroidism is indicated in most women with current or prior Graves' disease (discussed later).

Thionamide Therapy

ATDs are the mainstay of therapy for Graves' disease in pregnancy. PTU and methimazole (MMI), as well as its prodrug carbimazole, are equally effective in controlling hyperthyroidism during pregnancy, with a mean time to normalization of free T4 index of 7 to 8 weeks.[21] Both PTU and MMI cross the placenta and enter fetal circulation.[22,23] ATD therapy is associated with teratogenicity, with more severe defects seen with MMI than PTU. MMI embryopathy, which includes aplasia cutis, choanal atresia, esophageal atresia, umbilicocele, omphalomesenteric duct anomalies, ventricular septal defects, and dysmorphic facial features, is seen in 2% to 4% of children exposed to MMI in utero, particularly with exposure during gestational weeks 6 to 10.[24–27] Although PTU has been considered safe in pregnancy,[28–30] a population-based Danish study identified excess birth defects in 2% to 3% of children exposed to PTU, predominantly face and neck malformations (preauricular and branchial sinus/fistula/cyst) and urinary system malformations (renal cyst/hydronephrosis) in boys.[25,31] Although these defects are less severe than those seen with MMI, surgery was required for most of the children with urinary system malformations.[31]

In light of these considerations, when available, PTU is favored rather than MMI in the first trimester during organogenesis. However, the United States Food and Drug Administration (FDA) issued a black box warning for PTU in 2010 regarding the potential for fulminant hepatic failure; subsequently an advisory committee of the American Thyroid Association (ATA) and FDA jointly recommended limiting PTU to the first trimester.[28] The most recent practice guidelines of the ATA for the diagnosis and management of thyroid disease during pregnancy and postpartum deemed that no recommendation could be made regarding the appropriateness of switching agents after 16 weeks.[19] Should a change be made, the recommended conversion of MMI/PTU is a ratio of 1:20 for total daily dose (ie, 5 mg of MMI once daily to 50 mg of PTU twice a day).

Given the teratogenic effects of thionamides, use in pregnancy needs to be considered carefully. As a result of this, recent recommendations by both the ATA and the European Thyroid Association consider discontinuation of ATDs in early pregnancy altogether for low-risk patients (**Box 1**), identified as women on low doses of thionamides (MMI 5–10 mg/d or PTU 50–200 mg/d).[19,20] An important factor for decision making is the presence or absence of TRAb, noting that, in nonpregnant patients, less than 5% of patients with negative TRAb relapse within 8 weeks of discontinuing ATDs.[32] Other risk factors for relapse include duration of prior treatment less than 6 months, low or suppressed TSH levels on ATD therapy, and Graves' ophthalmopathy.[26,33] If ATDs are discontinued, thyroid function tests should be monitored every 1 to 2 weeks in the first trimester, and every 2 to 4 weeks in the second and third trimesters if the patient remains euthyroid.[19,20]

Box 1
Factors predicting successful withdrawal of antithyroid drugs in first trimester pregnancy

Low thionamide dose (MMI 5–10 mg/d or PTU 50–200 mg/d)

Serum TRAb undetectable/low level

Normal TSH levels

Duration of thionamide therapy longer than 6 months

No evidence of ophthalmopathy

When ATD therapy is needed in pregnancy, the lowest dose to control hyperthyroidism should be used. Fetal thyroid function is affected by both stimulatory effects of TRAb and inhibitory effects of ATDs. Maternal T4, but not T3 levels have been shown to strongly correlate with fetal T4 levels. Maintaining maternal free T4 levels in a mildly thyrotoxic range helps preserve a euthyroid fetal status.[34] Therapeutic targets are a free T4 level at the upper limit or moderately greater than the reference range, using pregnancy-specific reference ranges when available. Alternatively, a total T4 target of approximately 1.5 times the upper limit of normal of the nonpregnant reference range can be used in the second or third trimesters.[19] In the third trimester, about one-third of patients still requiring ATDs are able to have therapy discontinued because of disease remission.[35] Cessation of ATDs in the third trimester should be considered, particularly if TSH level is not suppressed and TRAb is undetectable. The use of ATDs is summarized in **Table 1**.

A block-and-replace strategy, in which ATDs are used in conjunction with levothyroxine therapy to render the mother euthyroid, should never be used to manage maternal Graves' disease in pregnancy. Both TRAb and ATDs readily cross the placenta, whereas levothyroxine passes the placenta to a limited degree. Although maternal thyroid function generally correlates with fetal thyroid function, a block-and-replace strategy may render the fetus hypothyroid and may cause fetal goiter.[36] An exception to this is in isolated fetal thyrotoxicosis when the mother is hypothyroid because of ablative therapy for Graves' disease with either surgery or radioiodine.

Beta-adrenergic Blockers

Beta blockage, specifically with propranolol, may be necessary to ameliorate the adrenergic symptoms of hyperthyroidism in early stages of disease before a euthyroid state is achieved. Long duration of β-blocker use has been associated with fetal bradycardia, neonatal hypoglycemia, and intrauterine growth restriction, so the shortest possible duration should be used.[37]

Iodides

Cases of congenital hypothyroidism caused by excess maternal iodine intake have been reported,[38] but low doses may be safe. A recent study substituted MMI with low-dose potassium iodine at a dose of 10 to 30 mg/d in the first trimester, with initiation at a median of 6 weeks gestation, and showed a lower incidence of congenital anomalies compared with ATD therapy and no evidence of neonatal thyroid dysfunction or goiter.[39] Although there are insufficient data to recommend this therapy, and results may not be generalizable outside of Japan, a country with high dietary iodine consumption, further study is warranted. Saturated solution of potassium iodide (SSKI) is indicated in preparation for surgery, as discussed later.

Surgery

Surgery for Graves' disease in pregnancy is generally avoided. Following surgery, TRAb levels decline slowly, with 70% to 80% of patients having disappearance of TRAb by 18 months[40]; therefore, in mothers requiring ATDs who subsequently undergo thyroidectomy in pregnancy, the risk of fetal thyrotoxicosis may persist.[36] Total thyroidectomy should be considered for women with severe hyperthyroidism and poor ATD compliance or inability to gain control with high-dose ATDs, allergies, or severe drug reactions for which ATDs are contraindicated, or with compressive goiter. The American College of Obstetricians and Gynecologists (ACOG) recommends performing surgery in the second trimester if feasible, because of fewer preterm contractions and less risk of spontaneous abortion, but also advises that a medically indicated

Table 1
Summary of antithyroid drug therapy in pregnancy[19]

First Trimester	Second Trimester	Third Trimester	All Trimesters
Consider stopping ATDs in low-risk patients (see **Box 1**) If ATDs d/c, monitor TFTs every 1–2 wk	If no ATDs, monitor TFTs every 2–4 wk if euthyroid	If no ATDs, monitor TFTs every 2–4 wk if euthyroid	—
If continued ATD therapy, change to PTU (MMI/PTU ratio of 1:20 for total daily dose)	If continued ATD therapy, consider changing from PTU to MMI after 16 wk gestational age	If continued ATD therapy, consider d/c ATDs if TRAb undetectable and TSH nonsuppressed	Monitor TFTs every 4 wk or sooner if indicated Use lowest available ATD dose to achieve free T4 at the upper limit or moderately above the reference range (pregnant if available) or total T4 target of ~1.5 times the upper limit of normal of the nonpregnant reference range

Abbreviations: d/c, discontinue; TFTs, thyroid function tests.

Data from Alexander EK, Pearce EN, Brent GA, et al. 2017 Guidelines of the American Thyroid Association for the Diagnosis and Management of Thyroid Disease During Pregnancy and the Postpartum. Thyroid 2017;27(3):315–89.

surgery should never be denied in any trimester of pregnancy.[41] If total thyroidectomy is performed in pregnancy, preoperative preparation with beta-blockade and SSKI (50–100 mg/d) are recommended.[19]

Radioactive Iodine

I-131 therapy is absolutely contraindicated in pregnancy; this may cross the placenta and cause permanent hypothyroidism because the developing fetus can concentrate I-131 starting at 10 weeks.[42] In addition, whole-body fetal irradiation can occur, from both transplacental passage of I-131 and external radiation from maternal tissues, particularly the bladder.[43]

MANAGEMENT OF TOXIC MULTINODULAR GOITER OR AUTONOMOUS NODULES

Functional thyroid nodules are uncommon in women less than 40 years of age.[44] Unlike Graves' disease, in which TRAb stimulates the fetal thyroid and ATDs block fetal thyroid hormone synthesis, ATDs for autonomous nodules are unopposed in fetal circulation, therefore the risk of fetal hypothyroidism and goiter may be greater. Because the degree of hyperthyroidism from autonomous nodules is typically milder than in Graves' disease, ATDs may not be required. Should ATDs be needed, careful monitoring and use of the lowest necessary dose to keep free/total T4 levels in the ranges described previously should occur, and the fetus should be monitored for signs of hypothyroidism and goiter.[19]

FETAL AND NEONATAL HYPERTHYROIDISM

Fetal and neonatal Graves' disease can complicate 1% to 5% of pregnancies in mothers with a current or prior history of Graves' disease, and is caused by transplacental passage of TRAb, which can stimulate fetal TSH receptors and alter fetal thyroid hormone production starting around 20 weeks gestation.[45,46]

Fetal thyrotoxicosis occurs in the fetus after 20 weeks gestation and can lead to goiter (**Fig. 1**), fetal tachycardia, growth restriction, advanced bone age, craniosynostosis (premature closing of cranial sutures), heart failure, nonimmune fetal hydrops, and intrauterine death.[45,47] Neonatal thyrotoxicosis is very likely when fetal hyperthyroidism is present, is transient, and generally resolves 4 to 6 months after birth following clearance of maternal TRAb. Signs and symptoms of neonatal hyperthyroidism include goiter, tachycardia, poor feeding, irritability, tremors, sweating, and difficulty sleeping. Proptosis, craniosynostosis, and microcephaly are sometimes seen. Without prompt treatment with antithyroid drugs, cardiac failure and death may occur.[48]

In order to identify pregnancies at risk for these conditions, TRAb levels should be monitored. Two types of assays are commercially available: immunoassays for TRAb are unable to differentiate between stimulating and inhibitory antibodies, whereas bioassays for thyroid-stimulating immunoglobulins (TSIs) are specific for antibodies that stimulate the TSH receptor. However, in the clinical scenario of active maternal Graves', the presence of TRAb by either assay is stimulatory.[49] TRAb by immunoassay is currently the recommended screening test to assess risk for fetal/neonatal Graves' disease. There are no data using TSI to further risk stratify TRAb-positive pregnancies for enhanced screening.[47]

TRAb should first be measured in early pregnancy in all women with active Graves' disease or with a prior history of Graves' disease treated with radioactive iodine or surgery. The ATA now recommends that women in biochemical remission of Graves' disease without prior history of definitive therapy do not require TRAb screening because

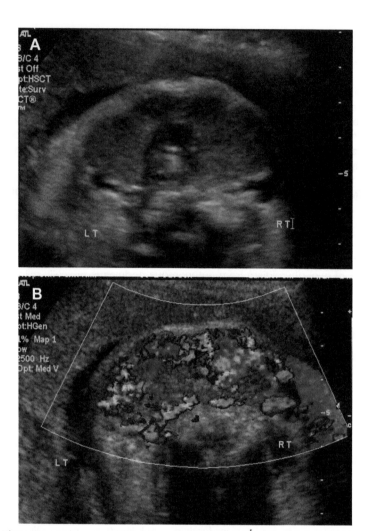

Fig. 1. Ultrasonography scan of fetal thyroid showing goiter (*A*) with increased vascularity (*B*) in a 32-week-old fetus with hyperthyroidism; fetal tachycardia and advanced bone age were also present.

of very low risk to the infant,[50] although the ETA continues to support screening of all women with a history of autoimmune thyroid disease.[20] If serum TRAb level is not increased in early pregnancy, no additional screening is necessary. Otherwise, TRAb should be measured at 18 to 22 weeks to screen for risk of fetal thyrotoxicosis, and, if increased, again at 30 to 34 weeks to assess for risk of neonatal thyrotoxicosis.

A TRAb measurement exceeding 3 times the upper limit of normal for the assay identifies at-risk pregnancies requiring further screening of the fetus and/or neonate. A recent meta-analysis of 20 studies including 53 cases of fetal and/or neonatal thyrotoxicosis supported this criterion. The lowest TRAb level associated with disease, measured by a second-generation immunoassay, was 4.4 U/L in the third trimester of pregnancy, which was 3.7 times the upper limit of normal.[47] In addition, all pregnancies in which uncontrolled maternal hyperthyroidism persists require fetal and neonatal screening. Fetal monitoring should include assessment of growth, heart rate, amniotic fluid volume, and thyroid ultrasonography to assess for goiter,[19] starting at 20 weeks and repeated every 4 to 6 weeks.[46]

Fetal thyroid ultrasonography has excellent sensitivity and specificity to detect clinically significant fetal thyroid disease.[19,51] However, goiter may occur from fetal hyperthyroidism caused by transplacental passage of TRAb, or because of the inhibitory effect of maternal ATD therapy leading to fetal hypothyroidism. Assessing the thyroid status of the mother clinically is a key indicator to help differentiate these two conditions. Fetal tachycardia and advanced fetal bone age also suggest hyperthyroidism. In select cases in which the diagnosis remains uncertain, umbilical cord blood sampling (cordocentesis) can be performed; however, this is invasive and carries a 0.5% to 2.0% risk of complications such as fetal infection, bleeding, bradycardia, preterm labor, and fetal death.[52–55] When fetal thyrotoxicosis is present and the mother is not on ATDs, such as in levothyroxine-replaced women with a history of prior radioiodine of surgery, ATDs can be given to the mother to treat the fetal hyperthyroidism while continuing the mother on levothyroxine. In cases of fetal goiter and hypothyroidism from maternal ATD therapy, symptoms may improve or resolve with dose reduction or discontinuation of maternal ATDs.[56–59]

Whenever neonatal hyperthyroidism is suspected, TRAb level should be measured in cord blood at delivery; nearly one-third of infants with increased cord blood TRAb levels develop neonatal hyperthyroidism. Maternal ATDs are metabolized by day of life 5 and most cases of neonatal hyperthyroidism present by 14 days of life.[48] A recent retrospective multicenter study of 280,000 births, including 415 women with Graves' disease, found that a TSH level of less than 0.9 mU/L between days 3 and 7 of life predicted neonatal hyperthyroidism with a sensitivity of 78% and specificity of 99%.[60]

LACTATION CONSIDERATIONS
Antithyroid Drugs

Small amounts of ATDs enter breastmilk. The use of ATDs in doses up to 20 mg/d of MMI or 450 mg/d of PTU, taken immediately following a feed, seems to be safe without affecting infant thyroid function, growth, or intelligence quotient.[19,61,62] No routine screening of the infant's thyroid function is recommended in the absence of abnormal growth or cognition. There are no reports of breastfed infants developing agranulocytosis or hepatotoxicity from ATDs.[61]

Radiopharmaceuticals

I-131 therapy is absolutely contraindicated during breastfeeding because it passes into breastmilk and has a long half-life; this poses risks of radiation exposure to the infant and maternal breast tissue, which concentrates radioiodine. Maternal weaning should occur at least 6 weeks before administration of I-131, although breastfeeding can be performed in subsequent pregnancies. Because of the shorter half-life of the isotope, I-123 scans can be performed during lactation, but it is recommended that breastmilk be pumped and discarded for 3 to 4 days following the test.[19] Tc-99m pertechnetate also passes into breastmilk, which can be pumped and discarded on the day of the test.[19]

REFERENCES

1. Glinoer D. Thyroid hyperfunction during pregnancy. Thyroid 1998;8(9):859–64.
2. Goodwin TM, Montoro M, Mestman JH. Transient hyperthyroidism and hyperemesis gravidarum: clinical aspects. Am J Obstet Gynecol 1992;167(3):648–52.

3. Tan JY, Loh KC, Yeo GS, et al. Transient hyperthyroidism of hyperemesis gravidarum. BJOG 2002;109(6):683–8.
4. Cooper DS, Laurberg P. Hyperthyroidism in pregnancy. Lancet Diabetes Endocrinol 2013;1(3):238–49.
5. Casey BM, Dashe JS, Wells CE, et al. Subclinical hyperthyroidism and pregnancy outcomes. Obstet Gynecol 2006;107(2 Pt 1):337–41.
6. Aggarawal N, Suri V, Singla R, et al. Pregnancy outcome in hyperthyroidism: a case control study. Gynecol Obstet Invest 2014;77(2):94–9.
7. Millar LK, Wing DA, Leung AS, et al. Low birth weight and preeclampsia in pregnancies complicated by hyperthyroidism. Obstet Gynecol 1994;84(6):946–9.
8. Sheffield JS, Cunningham FG. Thyrotoxicosis and heart failure that complicate pregnancy. Am J Obstet Gynecol 2004;190(1):211–7.
9. Glinoer D, De Nayer P, Robyn C, et al. Serum levels of intact human chorionic gonadotropin (HCG) and its free alpha and beta subunits, in relation to maternal thyroid stimulation during normal pregnancy. J Endocrinol Invest 1993;16(11):881–8.
10. Mori M, Amino N, Tamaki H, et al. Morning sickness and thyroid function in normal pregnancy. Obstet Gynecol 1988;72(3 Pt 1):355–9.
11. Grun JP, Meuris S, De Nayer P, et al. The thyrotrophic role of human chorionic gonadotrophin (hCG) in the early stages of twin (versus single) pregnancies. Clin Endocrinol 1997;46(6):719–25.
12. Patil-Sisodia K, Mestman JH. Graves' hyperthyroidism and pregnancy: a clinical update. Endocr Pract 2010;16(1):118–29.
13. Carle A, Knudsen N, Pedersen IB, et al. Determinants of serum T4 and T3 at the time of diagnosis in nosological types of thyrotoxicosis: a population-based study. Eur J Endocrinol 2013;169(5):537–45.
14. Andersen SL, Olsen J, Carle A, et al. Hyperthyroidism incidence fluctuates widely in and around pregnancy and is at variance with some other autoimmune diseases: a Danish population-based study. J Clin Endocrinol Metab 2015;100(3):1164–71.
15. Amino N, Tanizawa O, Mori H, et al. Aggravation of thyrotoxicosis in early pregnancy and after delivery in Graves' disease. J Clin Endocrinol Metab 1982;55(1):108–12.
16. Zakarija M, McKenzie JM. Pregnancy-associated changes in the thyroid-stimulating antibody of Graves' disease and the relationship to neonatal hyperthyroidism. J Clin Endocrinol Metab 1983;57(5):1036–40.
17. Amino N, Izumi Y, Hidaka Y, et al. No increase of blocking type anti-thyrotropin receptor antibodies during pregnancy in patients with Graves' disease. J Clin Endocrinol Metab 2003;88(12):5871–4.
18. Ide A, Amino N, Kang S, et al. Differentiation of postpartum Graves' thyrotoxicosis from postpartum destructive thyrotoxicosis using antithyrotropin receptor antibodies and thyroid blood flow. Thyroid 2014;24(6):1027–31.
19. Alexander EK, Pearce EN, Brent GA, et al. 2017 guidelines of the American Thyroid Association for the diagnosis and management of thyroid disease during pregnancy and the postpartum. Thyroid 2017;27(3):315–89.
20. Kahaly GJ, Bartalena L, Hegedus L, et al. 2018 European Thyroid Association guideline for the management of graves' hyperthyroidism. Eur Thyroid J 2018;7(4):167–86.
21. Wing DA, Millar LK, Koonings PP, et al. A comparison of propylthiouracil versus methimazole in the treatment of hyperthyroidism in pregnancy. Am J Obstet Gynecol 1994;170(1 Pt 1):90–5.

22. Gardner DF, Cruikshank DP, Hays PM, et al. Pharmacology of propylthiouracil (PTU) in pregnant hyperthyroid women: correlation of maternal PTU concentrations with cord serum thyroid function tests. J Clin Endocrinol Metab 1986; 62(1):217–20.
23. Mortimer RH, Cannell GR, Addison RS, et al. Methimazole and propylthiouracil equally cross the perfused human term placental lobule. J Clin Endocrinol Metab 1997;82(9):3099–102.
24. Yoshihara A, Noh J, Yamaguchi T, et al. Treatment of graves' disease with antithyroid drugs in the first trimester of pregnancy and the prevalence of congenital malformation. J Clin Endocrinol Metab 2012;97(7):2396–403.
25. Andersen SL, Olsen J, Wu CS, et al. Birth defects after early pregnancy use of antithyroid drugs: a Danish nationwide study. J Clin Endocrinol Metab 2013; 98(11):4373–81.
26. Laurberg P, Andersen SL. Therapy of endocrine disease: antithyroid drug use in early pregnancy and birth defects: time windows of relative safety and high risk? Eur J Endocrinol 2014;171(1):R13–20.
27. Seo GH, Kim TH, Chung JH. Antithyroid drugs and congenital malformations: a Nationwide Korean Cohort Study. Ann Intern Med 2018;168(6):405–13.
28. Bahn RS, Burch HS, Cooper DS, et al. The role of propylthiouracil in the management of Graves' disease in adults: report of a meeting jointly sponsored by the American Thyroid Association and the Food and Drug Administration. Thyroid 2009;19(7):673–4.
29. Rosenfeld H, Ornoy A, Shechtman S, et al. Pregnancy outcome, thyroid dysfunction and fetal goitre after in utero exposure to propylthiouracil: a controlled cohort study. Br J Clin Pharmacol 2009;68(4):609–17.
30. Clementi M, Di Gianantonio E, Cassina M, et al. Treatment of hyperthyroidism in pregnancy and birth defects. J Clin Endocrinol Metab 2010;95(11):E337–41.
31. Andersen SL, Olsen J, Wu CS, et al. Severity of birth defects after propylthiouracil exposure in early pregnancy. Thyroid 2014;24(10):1533–40.
32. Nedrebo BG, Holm PI, Uhlving S, et al. Predictors of outcome and comparison of different drug regimens for the prevention of relapse in patients with Graves' disease. Eur J Endocrinol 2002;147(5):583–9.
33. Laurberg P. Remission of Graves' disease during anti-thyroid drug therapy. Time to reconsider the mechanism? Eur J Endocrinol 2006;155(6):783–6.
34. Momotani N, Noh J, Oyanagi H, et al. Antithyroid drug therapy for Graves' disease during pregnancy. Optimal regimen for fetal thyroid status. N Engl J Med 1986;315(1):24–8.
35. Hamburger JI. Diagnosis and management of Graves' disease in pregnancy. Thyroid 1992;2(3):219–24.
36. Laurberg P, Bournaud C, Karmisholt J, et al. Management of Graves' hyperthyroidism in pregnancy: focus on both maternal and foetal thyroid function, and caution against surgical thyroidectomy in pregnancy. Eur J Endocrinol 2009; 160(1):1–8.
37. Rubin PC. Current concepts: beta-blockers in pregnancy. N Engl J Med 1981; 305(22):1323–6.
38. Connelly KJ, Boston BA, Pearce EN, et al. Congenital hypothyroidism caused by excess prenatal maternal iodine ingestion. J Pediatr 2012;161(4):760–2.
39. Yoshihara A, Noh JY, Watanabe N, et al. Substituting potassium iodide for methimazole as the treatment for Graves' disease during the first trimester may reduce the incidence of congenital anomalies: a retrospective study at a single medical institution in Japan. Thyroid 2015;25(10):1155–61.

40. Laurberg P, Wallin G, Tallstedt L, et al. TSH-receptor autoimmunity in Graves' disease after therapy with anti-thyroid drugs, surgery, or radioiodine: a 5-year prospective randomized study. Eur J Endocrinol 2008;158(1):69–75.

41. Committee opinion no. 696: nonobstetric surgery during pregnancy. Obstet Gynecol 2017;129(4):777–8.

42. Bural GG, Laymon CM, Mountz JM. Nuclear imaging of a pregnant patient: should we perform nuclear medicine procedures during pregnancy? Mol Imaging Radionucl Ther 2012;21(1):1–5.

43. International Atomic Energy Agency. Radiation protection of pregnant women in nuclear medicine 2018. Available at: https://www.iaea.org/resources/rpop/health-professionals/nuclear-medicine/pregnant-women#6. Accessed November 17, 2018.

44. Carle A, Pedersen IB, Knudsen N, et al. Epidemiology of subtypes of hyperthyroidism in Denmark: a population-based study. Eur J Endocrinol 2011;164(5): 801–9.

45. Zimmerman D. Fetal and neonatal hyperthyroidism. Thyroid 1999;9(7):727–33.

46. Leger J. Management of fetal and neonatal Graves' disease. Horm Res Paediatr 2017;87(1):1–6.

47. van Dijk MM, Smits IH, Fliers E, et al. Maternal thyrotropin receptor antibody concentration and the risk of fetal and neonatal thyrotoxicosis: a systematic review. Thyroid 2018;28(2):257–64.

48. Samuels SL, Namoc SM, Bauer AJ. Neonatal thyrotoxicosis. Clin Perinatol 2018; 45(1):31–40.

49. Mortimer RH, Tyack SA, Galligan JP, et al. Graves' disease in pregnancy: TSH receptor binding inhibiting immunoglobulins and maternal and neonatal thyroid function. Clin Endocrinol 1990;32(2):141–52.

50. Laurberg P, Nygaard B, Glinoer D, et al. Guidelines for TSH-receptor antibody measurements in pregnancy: results of an evidence-based symposium organized by the European Thyroid Association. Eur J Endocrinol 1998;139(6):584–6.

51. Luton D, Le Gac I, Vuillard E, et al. Management of Graves' disease during pregnancy: the key role of fetal thyroid gland monitoring. J Clin Endocrinol Metab 2005;90(11):6093–8.

52. Boupaijit K, Wanapirak C, Piyamongkol W, et al. Effect of placenta penetration during cordocentesis at mid-pregnancy on fetal outcomes. Prenat Diagn 2012; 32(1):83–7.

53. Porreco RP, Bloch CA. Fetal blood sampling in the management of intrauterine thyrotoxicosis. Obstet Gynecol 1990;76(3 Pt 2):509–12.

54. Weiner CP. Cordocentesis for diagnostic indications: two years' experience. Obstet Gynecol 1987;70(4):664–8.

55. Weiner CP, Wenstrom KD, Sipes SL, et al. Risk factors for cordocentesis and fetal intravascular transfusion. Am J Obstet Gynecol 1991;165(4 Pt 1):1020–5.

56. Cheron RG, Kaplan MM, Larsen PR, et al. Neonatal thyroid function after propylthiouracil therapy for maternal Graves' disease. N Engl J Med 1981;304(9): 525–8.

57. Polak M, Le Gac I, Vuillard E, et al. Fetal and neonatal thyroid function in relation to maternal Graves' disease. Best Pract Res Clin Endocrinol Metab 2004;18(2): 289–302.

58. Cohen O, Pinhas-Hamiel O, Sivan E, et al. Serial in utero ultrasonographic measurements of the fetal thyroid: a new complementary tool in the management of maternal hyperthyroidism in pregnancy. Prenat Diagn 2003;23(9):740–2.

59. Ochoa-Maya MR, Frates MC, Lee-Parritz A, et al. Resolution of fetal goiter after discontinuation of propylthiouracil in a pregnant woman with Graves' hyperthyroidism. Thyroid 1999;9(11):1111–4.
60. Banige M, Polak M, Luton D. Prediction of neonatal hyperthyroidism. J Pediatr 2018;197:249–54.e1.
61. Mandel SJ, Cooper DS. The use of antithyroid drugs in pregnancy and lactation. J Clin Endocrinol Metab 2001;86(6):2354–9.
62. Azizi F, Khoshniat M, Bahrainian M, et al. Thyroid function and intellectual development of infants nursed by mothers taking methimazole. J Clin Endocrinol Metab 2000;85(9):3233–8.

Hypothyroidism in Pregnancy

Peter N. Taylor, PhD*, John H. Lazarus, MD

KEYWORDS

• Hypothyroidism • Pregnancy • Levothyroxine • Screening • TPO • Iodine

KEY POINTS

- Hypothyroidism is common in women of child-bearing age and commonly associated with adverse obstetric and offspring outcomes.
- Pregnancy places substantial additional demands on the thyroid axis and women who have normal thyroid function before pregnancy may have insufficient reserve for pregnancy, especially those with autoimmune thyroid disease.
- Levothyroxine is the treatment of hypothyroidism; in women established on levothyroxine before pregnancy doses usually need increasing.
- Screening for thyroid disease in pregnancy is being undertaken in some countries, although this is a major debate in thyroidology at present.

INTRODUCTION

Adequate thyroid hormone is essential for maintaining a pregnancy and optimal fetal development.[1] During the first half of pregnancy, the fetus is entirely dependent on maternal thyroid hormone. Thyroid disorders, particularly low thyroid function, is common in women of childbearing age and frequently encountered in antenatal clinics. It is well established that overt hypothyroidism results in substantially higher risks of adverse pregnancy and offspring outcomes and all endocrine and obstetric societies recommend treating this. Iodine is essential for thyroid hormone production, so adequacy here is vital during pregnancy and in women of reproductive age. There is now increasing evidence that even borderline thyroid function and thyroid autoimmunity are also associated with adverse outcomes raising the possibility that universal thyroid screening in pregnancy should be considered.[2] Furthermore, pregnancy places additional demands on the thyroid axis, so women with adequate thyroid hormone before pregnancy may fail to meet the additional demands of pregnancy.

Clinically thyroid function is assessed by measuring the pituitary hormone thyroid-stimulating hormone (TSH) and thyroid hormone levels. The complex inverse

Disclosure Statement: No conflicts of interest to disclose.
Thyroid Research Group, Systems Immunity Research Institute, Cardiff University School of Medicine, UHW, C2 Link Corridor, Heath Park, Cardiff CF14 4XN, UK
* Corresponding author.
E-mail address: taylorpn@cardiff.ac.uk

Endocrinol Metab Clin N Am 48 (2019) 547–556
https://doi.org/10.1016/j.ecl.2019.05.010
0889-8529/19/© 2019 Elsevier Inc. All rights reserved.
endo.theclinics.com

relationship between TSH and thyroid hormone results in small changes in thyroid hormone levels causing larger changes in TSH. It is essential to measure thyroid hormone levels and TSH to differentiate between overt and subclinical thyroid disease.

IODINE STATUS AND THYROID FUNCTION

Iodine is essential for the synthesis of thyroid hormones.[3] The recommended daily iodine intake in pregnancy has recently been increased to 250 μg/d, which implies a urinary iodine excretion of 150 to 250 μg/d as being adequate.[4,5] Iodine deficiency during pregnancy is associated with maternal goiter and results eventually in a reduced circulating maternal thyroxine concentration. These effects are preventable by iodine supplementation[6] and benefits of this are observed in areas of severe iodine deficiency (24-hour urinary iodine <50 μg) and in areas of mild to moderate deficiency.[7] Children born to mothers with profound iodine deficiency show impaired neurointellectual development, sometimes to the extreme of cretinism in severely deficient states. These effects are reduced by iodine administration before and even during gestation and this should be performed in areas of moderate to severe iodine deficiency.[3] It is noteworthy that even mild-moderate iodine deficiency in pregnant women is associated with adverse maternal effects including goiter[8] and lower intelligence quotient (IQ) in offspring.[9] Although a recent trial did not show benefit on iodine supplementation during pregnancy in areas of mild iodine deficiency[10] further studies are required. Assessment of iodine status is challenging and urinary iodine remains an imperfect marker of iodine status; serum thyroglobulin may become a useful biomarker of iodine status. Endocrine disruptors, such as perchlorate, may exacerbate iodine deficiency and may also have a deleterious effect on offspring neurodevelopment.[11,12]

IMPACT OF PREGNANCY ON THE MATERNAL THYROID STATUS

Pregnancy places substantial demands on the maternal thyroid axis, and these are summarized in **Table 1** and **Fig. 1**. The fetal thyroid is not functional until 18 to 20 weeks gestation, so additional maternal thyroid hormone is required to meet this demand. Additionally, there is increased thyroxine binding globulin and increased thyroid hormone degradation by placental type 3 deiodinase,[13] which also increases demands. There is also increased urinary iodine excretion during pregnancy. Urinary iodine excretion in pregnancy is maximal in the first trimester, followed by a decline in the second and third trimesters. It is increasingly recognized that countries may have iodine sufficiency in the general population, but be insufficient for pregnancy, the United Kingdom and Russia are notable examples of this.[14] This iodine deficiency can result in increased risk of maternal goiter and hypothyroidism. The pregnancy hormone human chorionic gonadotrophin (hCG) does stimulate the thyroid to produce thyroid hormone, which assists with meeting the increased demands on the thyroid axis in pregnancy. Recent data suggest that thyroid peroxidase (TPO) antibody (TPOAb)-positive women may have an impaired thyroidal response to hCG[15] and therefore may not meet the additional demands at key points over pregnancy. This may explain at least in part why women with thyroid autoimmunity with positive TPOAb have increased risk of adverse obstetric outcomes, which is independent of thyroid status.

ASSESSMENT OF THYROID STATUS DURING PREGNANCY

It is important to recognize that assessment of thyroid function in pregnancy is more complex than in the general adult population. The previously mentioned physiologic

Table 1		
Physiologic changes that influence thyroid function in pregnancy		
Physiologic Change	**Effect on Thyroid Function Test Results**	**Impact on Interpretation of Thyroid Function Tests**
↑ Thyroxine-binding globulin	↑ Serum total T3 and T4 concentrations	Total thyroid hormone levels may be misleading; need to rely on free thyroid hormone levels.
↑ Human chorionic gonadotrophin secretion	↑ Free T4 and ↓ TSH	High human chorionic gonadotrophin levels may result in gestational thyrotoxicosis. This usually only requires symptomatic treatment but needs to be distinguished from pathologic thyroid disease. Response possibly impaired in TPO antibody–positive women.
↑ Iodine excretion	↓ Thyroid hormone production in iodine-deficient areas	Need to be mindful of iodine deficiency and ensure optimal intake ideally before conception.
↑ Plasma volume	↑ T3 and T4 pool size	
Increased type 3 5-deiodinase (inner ring deiodination) activity from the placental	↑ T3 and T4 degradation	May explain in part the increasing thyroid demand in pregnancy.
Thyroid enlargement (in some women)	Increased thyroglobulin	Small goiters is common in pregnancy, but may be a sign of low thyroid function so merits thyroid function testing.

Adapted from Lazarus JH. Thyroid function in pregnancy. Br Med Bull. 2011;97:137-48. https://doi.org/10.1093/bmb/ldq039. Epub 2010 Dec 23; with permission.

changes in pregnancy have a substantial effect on the interpretation of thyroid function tests in pregnancy and result in a downward shift of TSH reference intervals. A pragmatic upper limit of 2.5 mU/L was previously advocated for TSH but recent data now show this threshold to be too low.[16] One approach suggested in the current guidelines of the American Thyroid Association (ATA) is to set the pregnancy reference range at 0.5 mU/L and 0.4 mU/L less than the upper and lower nonpregnant reference range, respectively, reflecting the anticipated magnitude of the TSH drop.[17]

Current ATA guidelines advocate the use of pregnancy-specific, local population-based reference ranges where possible[17]; however, it is well recognized that such data are not widely available. Assessment of thyroid function in pregnancy is also best done according to pregnancy-specific reference ranges calculated in a population of pregnant women free of key factors that interfere with thyroid function including women with known thyroid disease (including thyroid autoimmunity), use of thyroid-altering medication, known iodine deficiency, and high hCG states (twin pregnancies or in vitro fertilization conception). However, it is also well established that normal thyroid status changes over pregnancy and accurate classification of thyroid function in pregnant women requires the use of gestational age–specific reference ranges.[18] There is also growing evidence that specific reference ranges may be considered based on ethnicity,[19] body mass index,[20] and parity.[20]

With respect to FT4, the most commonly used immunoassays are prone to biases in pregnancy because of changes in thyroid-binding globulin and albumin

Physiological changes   Impact

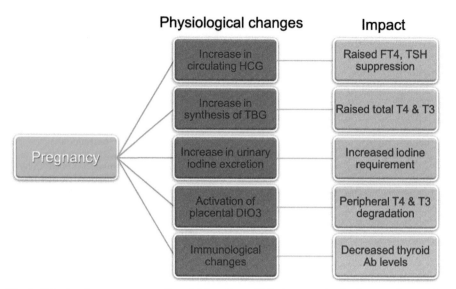

Fig. 1. Effects of pregnancy on thyroid function. HCG, human chorionic gonadotrophin; TBG, thyroid binding globulin.

concentrations.[17,21] Total T4 is a more predictable alternative because it typically rises by 50% of baseline values attaining peak levels by 16 weeks gestation.[17] However, total T4 is less clearly associated with adverse outcomes, so many clinicians prefer the use of FT4. More robust methods, such as equilibrium dialysis, liquid chromatography–tandem mass spectrometry, or FT4 index calculations, are cumbersome to perform and not routinely used.[17]

CLASSIFICATION AND EPIDEMIOLOGY OF THYROID ABNORMALITIES

Overt hypothyroidism in pregnancy is defined as a TSH level greater than the pregnancy-specific reference range and a low level of FT4. Although women established on levothyroxine make up around 1% of pregnancies, newly diagnosed overt hypothyroidism occurs in approximately 0.2% to 0.6% of pregnant women.[16,22] Treatment is mandatory because it is associated with profound adverse obstetric and offspring development outcomes. The milder forms of low thyroid dysfunction are subclinical hypothyroidism (TSH greater than the population's pregnancy reference range, but normal FT4) and isolated hypothyroxinemia (IH; normal TSH with FT4 in the lowest 2.5% of the reference range), and these are more common. Subclinical hypothyroidism with an elevated TSH and normal FT4 concentrations can occur in up to 18% of pregnancies depending on the precise definition and TSH assay used. Observational studies have indicated that subclinical hypothyroidism is associated with adverse pregnancy outcomes, but not offspring neurodevelopment. In contrast IH is associated with adverse outcomes with regard to offspring IQ and behavior, but less consistent associations have been observed for pregnancy outcomes.

Overt Hypothyroidism

Overt hypothyroidism has been repeatedly associated with substantial adverse impacts on obstetric outcomes and fetal neurodevelopment. Adverse obstetric outcomes include fetal loss, premature delivery, low birthweight, and preeclampisa.[22,23]

A large case-control study demonstrated that overt hypothyroidism resulted in a seven-point lower IQ in the offspring than in the children of women with normal thyroid function.[24] It is worth noting that women with adequately treated hypothyroidism have no higher risk of pregnancy complications, unlike those with untreated hypothyroidism, indicating that thyroid status is a clearly reversible risk factor for adverse obstetric outcomes.

Subclinical Hypothyroidism

Numerous studies have identified that subclinical hypothyroidism is associated with adverse pregnancy outcomes similar to what is seen with overt hypothyroidism but risk effects are more marginal. From meta-analyses of subclinical hypothyroidism the odds of the following outcomes were all statistically significant for adverse outcomes with 95% confidence intervals (CI) provided: miscarriage odds ratio (OR) = 1.90 (95% CI, 1.59–2.27) and OR = 2.01 (95% CI, 1.66–2.44), preterm delivery OR = 1.20 (95% CI, 0.97–1.50), growth restriction OR = 1.40 (95% CI, 0.64–2.80), preeclampsia OR = 1.70 (95% CI, 1.10–2.64), and gestational diabetes OR = 1.40 (95% CI, 0.64–2.80).[25] One problem with these analyses is that many studies have defined subclinical hypothyroidism differently. What is clear is that subclinical hypothyroidism does not seem to be associated with adverse neurobehavioral outcomes in the offspring.

Isolated Hypothyroxinemia

IH was originally considered to be a pregnancy-specific disease, reflecting a state of mild iodine deficiency. However, this has now been called into question because it also occurs in iodine-sufficient areas. Other risk factors for IH include iron status, body mass index, and placental angiogenic factors.[1] IH has been associated with impaired offspring developmental outcomes[26] and has also been associated with offspring verbal delay,[27] autism,[28] and attention-deficit/hyperactivity disorder.[29] In contrast to subclinical hypothyroidism it has not been consistently associated with adverse obstetric outcomes.

Thyroid Autoimmunity

Anti-TPOAb are found in around 10% of otherwise normal pregnant women. They are a marker of thyroid autoimmunity and the main risk factor for thyroid dysfunction in pregnancy and in the postpartum period. Even in euthyroid women TPOAb positivity is associated with premature delivery and fetal loss, although the exact mechanism remains unclear.[30,31] One randomized, controlled trial has shown that levothyroxine administration reduced the risk of fetal loss and premature delivery in euthyroid TPOAb-positive women.[32] A later study failed to replicate the benefits for fetal loss but did find a reduction in preterm delivery.[33] Women who are TPOAb-positive are at an increased risk of thyroid-related adverse pregnancy outcomes; the interaction of TPOAb positivity with higher TSH levels means it is likely that this risk is substantially increased in individuals who also have elevated TSH levels or those in the higher end of the normal range. Recently the TABLET trial showed no clear benefit of levothyroxine in euthyroid women with TPOAb positivity with regard to rate of live births.[34]

TRIALS OF TREATMENT WITH LEVOTHYROXINE IN WOMEN WITH BORDERLINE THYROID FUNCTION

All endocrine and obstetric societies recommend treating overt hypothyroidism in pregnancy, although there have been no recent trials in this area and to have a control group here is unethical. To date three large randomized controlled trials have investigated the effects of screening for and treating borderline low thyroid function in pregnancy: these are the Controlled Antenatal Thyroid Screening (CATS) study,[35] a study by Casey and colleagues,[36] and a recent study by Nazarpour and colleagues.[33] These trials are summarized in **Table 2**. The Nazarpour trial focused on preterm delivery and identified that levothyroxine may reduce the risk of preterm delivery in individuals with TSH levels greater than 4.0 mU/L (relative risk, 0.38; 95% CI, 0.15–0.98; $P = .04$).[33] Offspring IQ was not assessed in this study. The two other large randomized controlled trials, CATS[35] and the study by Casey and colleagues,[36] studied the effects of screening and treating borderline low thyroid function in pregnancy on offspring IQ and pregnancy outcomes. Neither study showed any beneficial effects of treatment on offspring IQ.[35,36] Reasons for failure to establish benefit aside from no treatment benefit, include the late initiation of treatment (particularly in the Casey study) and early age of IQ assessment (particularly in the CATS study). It is worth highlighting that neurologic development is crucial in the first 12 weeks of pregnancy. Follow on analysis of the CATS study revealed no apparent benefit of treatment at age 9 years, although this was only performed in a subset. Work in the follow-up CATS study also identified levothyroxine overtreatment may increase the risk of autism symptoms.[37] More recent analysis using data linkage and most of the CATS cohort (to include those with normal thyroid function) identified that levothyroxine treatment significantly reduced the risk of miscarriage/still birth.[37] Similarly, another prospective study did identify that

Table 2
Summary of trials correcting borderline low thyroid function

	CATS	Casey	Nazarpour
Year	2012	2017	2018
Countries in trial	United Kingdom, Italy	United States	Iran
Number with low thyroid function randomized	794	677	366
Placebo-controlled	No	Yes	No
Gestational age at recruitment (wk)	Median (IQR) Screening 12.3 (11.6–13.6) Controls 12.3 (11.6–13.5)	Mean (SD) Screening 16.6 (3.0) Controls 16.7 (3.0)	Mean (SD) Screening 11.4 (4.1) Controls 12.2 (4.3)
Baseline TSH mU/L	Median (IQR) Screening United Kingdom 3.8 (1.5–4.7) Screening Italy 3.1 (1.3–4.0) Controls United Kingdom 3.2 (1.2–4.2) Controls Italy 2.4 (1.3–3.9)	Mean (95% CI) Screening 4.5 (4.4–4.7) Controls 4.3 (4.2–4.5)	Median (IQR) Screening 3.8 (2.8–4.8)
Outcomes assessed	IQ age 3, IQ age 9 Obstetric outcomes (analyzed later and only in UK participants)	Pregnancy outcomes, offspring IQ and behavior	Preterm delivery
Benefit of levothyroxine	No benefit with regard to IQ Potential reduction in fetal loss	No benefits observed with regard to pregnancy outcomes and offspring IQ	May reduce preterm delivery at TSH levels >4.0 mU/L

Abbreviations: IQR, interquartile range; SD, standard deviation.

levothyroxine reduced the risk of miscarriage and preterm birth.[32] However, no benefit was observed with levothyroxine on obstetric outcomes in the Casey study, although again this may be caused by the late initiation of treatment.[36]

TREATMENT OF ESTABLISHED HYPOTHYROIDISM IN PREGNANCY

Approximately 1% of pregnant women are established on levothyroxine before pregnancy. In women established on levothyroxine before pregnancy, initial control in pregnancy is often suboptimal[38] and may be associated with increased odds of fetal loss[38]; therefore, optimization should ideally occur before conception.[39] Women of child-bearing age on levothyroxine should be reminded to increase their preconception dose of levothyroxine by 30% to 50% as soon as pregnancy is confirmed. One approach is to take double their usual levothyroxine dose on 2 days of the week.[40] It is worth noting, that dose increases needed are often higher in postsurgical or postablative hypothyroidism. Women on levothyroxine should also be aware of important drug interactions with iron supplements and proton pump inhibitors, which can impair levothyroxine absorption. Other drugs to be aware of that increase levothyroxine clearance include carbamazepine, rifampicin, and valproate. If overt hypothyroidism is diagnosed for the first time in pregnancy, we recommend starting a weight-based dose of 2 µg/kg/day.

Close monitoring of thyroid function is essential in pregnancy. We recommend checking thyroid function early in the first trimester and every 4 to 6 weeks thereafter. One should ideally aim for a TSH less than 2.5 mU/L in the first trimester and less than 3 mU/L in later pregnancy. One should aim to ensure that the FT4 level is not too high and aim for the upper half of the reference range. There is some evidence that over-replacement with levothyroxine may increase attention-deficit/hyperactivity symptoms and the relationship of FT4 and IQ is "U shaped" with low-normal and high-normal FT4 are associated with lower IQ.[26] After delivery we suggest returning levothyroxine to preconception dose and to recheck thyroid function at 6 weeks postpartum.

SCREENING FOR AND TREATING LOW THYROID FUNCTION IN PREGNANCY

Universal thyroid screening in pregnancy remains contentious.[2] It is noteworthy that screening for and treating low thyroid function meets almost all the screening criteria laid down by Wilson and Jungner.[41] In particular it is an important asymptomatic health problem, with an accepted treatment and a suitable diagnostic test. It is also economically viable.[42] However, at present it is still unclear what TSH threshold should be used for treatment in pregnancy and whether there should be a differential threshold based on TPO status. The criterion "there should be an agreed policy on who to treat" is therefore not met. However, because there is widespread variation in clinical practice at present, this should not necessarily prevent the introduction of universal thyroid screening and indeed regular audit and review may establish more definitive treatment thresholds. Current ATA guidance takes into account the potential for interaction by TPOAb status in its guidance, but did not recommended for or against universal thyroid screening.[17] This has not prevented some countries including Spain, China, and Poland from implementing universal thyroid screening. It is, however, accepted that targeted screening should be performed in those women at high risk for thyroid disease.[17,43] Women deemed at high risk for thyroid disease in pregnancy include those with previous thyroid disease; a visible goiter; symptoms suggestive of hypothyroidism or hyperthyroidism; those with a family history of thyroid disease; those with a history of type 1 diabetes or other autoimmune conditions including positive thyroid antibodies; and women with a previous history of infertility, fetal loss, or infertility. However, this targeted approach would miss approximately one-third of women with significant thyroid dysfunction.[44] This high-risk screening approach has been further called into question, because universal thyroid screening in pregnancy seems to be cost-effective; screening solely for overt hypothyroidism also had a cost-effectiveness ratio of $6776 per quality-adjusted life-year (QALY),[42] which is favorable compared with gestational diabetes mellitus screening ($12,078 per QALY) and is substantially less than the $50,000 per QALY figure used in the United States as a criterion for screening decisions. This work also indicated universal screening seems to be more cost-effective than targeted screening.

SUMMARY

Despite the dramatic recent advances in knowledge of thyroid physiology in pregnancy and the consequences of its variation, further research is required, in particular, prospective trials of early screening of thyroid function in pregnancy with obstetric and developmental outcomes assessed. Continued advocacy of iodine sufficiency in pregnancy and assessment of endocrine disruptors are also needed. In current practice monitoring of thyroid function in early pregnancy needs urgent optimization.

REFERENCES

1. Korevaar TIM, Medici M, Visser TJ, et al. Thyroid disease in pregnancy: new insights in diagnosis and clinical management. Nat Rev Endocrinol 2017;13(10): 610–22.
2. Taylor PN, Zouras S, Min T, et al. Thyroid screening in early pregnancy: pros and cons. Front Endocrinol (Lausanne) 2018;9:626.
3. Zimmermann MB. Iodine deficiency. Endocr Rev 2009;30(4):376–408.
4. Zimmermann MB, Gizak M, Abbott K, et al. Iodine deficiency in pregnant women in Europe. Lancet Diabetes Endocrinol 2015;3(9):672–4.
5. Taylor P, Vaidya B. Iodine supplementation in pregnancy: is it time? Clin Endocrinol (Oxf) 2016;85(1):10–4.
6. Zimmermann MB. Iodine deficiency in pregnancy and the effects of maternal iodine supplementation on the offspring: a review. Am J Clin Nutr 2009;89(2): 668S–72S.
7. Taylor PN, Okosieme OE, Dayan CM, et al. Therapy of endocrine disease: impact of iodine supplementation in mild-to-moderate iodine deficiency: systematic review and meta-analysis. Eur J Endocrinol 2014;170(1):R1–15.
8. Taylor PN, Razvi S, Pearce SH, et al. A review of the clinical consequences of variation in thyroid function within the reference range. J Clin Endocrinol Metab 2013; 98(9):3562–71.
9. Bath SC, Steer CD, Golding J, et al. Effect of inadequate iodine status in UK pregnant women on cognitive outcomes in their children: results from the Avon Longitudinal Study of Parents and Children (ALSPAC). Lancet 2013;382(9889):331–7.
10. Gowachirapant S, Jaiswal N, Melse-Boonstra A, et al. Effect of iodine supplementation in pregnant women on child neurodevelopment: a randomised, double-blind, placebo-controlled trial. Lancet Diabetes Endocrinol 2017;5(11):853–63.
11. Bellanger M, Demeneix B, Grandjean P, et al. Neurobehavioral deficits, diseases, and associated costs of exposure to endocrine-disrupting chemicals in the European Union. J Clin Endocrinol Metab 2015;100(4):1256–66.
12. Taylor PN, Okosieme OE, Murphy R, et al. Maternal perchlorate levels in women with borderline thyroid function during pregnancy and the cognitive development

of their offspring: data from the Controlled Antenatal Thyroid Study. J Clin Endocrinol Metab 2014;99(11):4291–8.

13. Brent GA. Maternal thyroid function: interpretation of thyroid function tests in pregnancy. Clin Obstet Gynecol 1997;40(1):3–15.

14. Taylor PN, Albrecht D, Scholz A, et al. Global epidemiology of hyperthyroidism and hypothyroidism. Nat Rev Endocrinol 2018;14(5):301–16.

15. Korevaar TI, Steegers EA, Pop VJ, et al. Thyroid autoimmunity impairs the thyroidal response to human chorionic gonadotropin: two population-based prospective cohort studies. J Clin Endocrinol Metab 2017;102(1):69–77.

16. Medici M, Korevaar TI, Visser WE, et al. Thyroid function in pregnancy: what is normal? Clin Chem 2015;61(5):704–13.

17. Alexander EK, Pearce EN, Brent GA, et al. 2017 guidelines of the American Thyroid Association for the diagnosis and management of thyroid disease during pregnancy and the postpartum. Thyroid 2017;27(3):315–89.

18. Stricker R, Echenard M, Eberhart R, et al. Evaluation of maternal thyroid function during pregnancy: the importance of using gestational age-specific reference intervals. Eur J Endocrinol 2007;157(4):509–14.

19. Korevaar TI, Medici M, de Rijke YB, et al. Ethnic differences in maternal thyroid parameters during pregnancy: the Generation R study. J Clin Endocrinol Metab 2013;98(9):3678–86.

20. Korevaar TI, de Rijke YB, Chaker L, et al. Stimulation of thyroid function by human chorionic gonadotropin during pregnancy: a risk factor for thyroid disease and a mechanism for known risk factors. Thyroid 2017;27(3):440–50.

21. Ross DS, Burch HB, Cooper DS, et al. 2016 American Thyroid Association guidelines for diagnosis and management of hyperthyroidism and other causes of thyrotoxicosis. Thyroid 2016;26(10):1343–421.

22. Krassas GE, Poppe K, Glinoer D. Thyroid function and human reproductive health. Endocr Rev 2010;31(5):702–55.

23. van den Boogaard E, Vissenberg R, Land JA, et al. Significance of (sub)clinical thyroid dysfunction and thyroid autoimmunity before conception and in early pregnancy: a systematic review. Hum Reprod Update 2011;17(5):605–19.

24. Haddow JE, Palomaki GE, Allan WC, et al. Maternal thyroid deficiency during pregnancy and subsequent neuropsychological development of the child. N Engl J Med 1999;341(8):549–55.

25. Velasco I, Taylor P. Identifying and treating subclinical thyroid dysfunction in pregnancy: emerging controversies. Eur J Endocrinol 2018;178(1):D1–12.

26. Korevaar TI, Muetzel R, Medici M, et al. Association of maternal thyroid function during early pregnancy with offspring IQ and brain morphology in childhood: a population-based prospective cohort study. Lancet Diabetes Endocrinol 2016; 4(1):35–43.

27. Henrichs J, Bongers-Schokking JJ, Schenk JJ, et al. Maternal thyroid function during early pregnancy and cognitive functioning in early childhood: the generation R study. J Clin Endocrinol Metab 2010;95(9):4227–34.

28. Román GC, Ghassabian A, Bongers-Schokking JJ, et al. Association of gestational maternal hypothyroxinemia and increased autism risk. Ann Neurol 2013; 74(5):733–42.

29. Vermiglio F, Lo Presti VP, Moleti M, et al. Attention deficit and hyperactivity disorders in the offspring of mothers exposed to mild-moderate iodine deficiency: a possible novel iodine deficiency disorder in developed countries. J Clin Endocrinol Metab 2004;89(12):6054–60.

30. Korevaar TI, Schalekamp-Timmermans S, de Rijke YB, et al. Hypothyroxinemia and TPO-antibody positivity are risk factors for premature delivery: the generation R study. J Clin Endocrinol Metab 2013;98(11):4382–90.

31. Thangaratinam S, Tan A, Knox E, et al. Association between thyroid autoantibodies and miscarriage and preterm birth: meta-analysis of evidence. BMJ 2011;342:d2616.

32. Negro R, Formoso G, Mangieri T, et al. Levothyroxine treatment in euthyroid pregnant women with autoimmune thyroid disease: effects on obstetrical complications. J Clin Endocrinol Metab 2006;91(7):2587–91.

33. Nazarpour S, Ramezani Tehrani F, Simbar M, et al. Effects of levothyroxine treatment on pregnancy outcomes in pregnant women with autoimmune thyroid disease. Eur J Endocrinol 2017;176(2):253–65.

34. Dhillon-Smith RK, Middleton LJ, Sunner KK, et al. Levothyroxine in women with thyroid peroxidase antibodies before conception. N Engl J Med 2019;380(14): 1316–25.

35. Lazarus JH, Bestwick JP, Channon S, et al. Antenatal thyroid screening and childhood cognitive function. N Engl J Med 2012;366(6):493–501.

36. Casey BM, Thom EA, Peaceman AM, et al. Treatment of subclinical hypothyroidism or hypothyroxinemia in pregnancy. N Engl J Med 2017;376(9):815–25.

37. Bartalena L, Fliers E, Hellen N, et al. Meeting abstracts from the 64th British Thyroid Association Annual Meeting. Thyroid Res 2017;10(1):2.

38. Taylor PN, Minassian C, Rehman A, et al. TSH levels and risk of miscarriage in women on long-term levothyroxine: a community-based study. J Clin Endocrinol Metab 2014;99(10):3895–902, jc20141954.

39. Okosieme OE, Khan I, Taylor PN. Preconception management of thyroid dysfunction. Clin Endocrinol (Oxf) 2018;89(3):269–79.

40. Yassa L, Marqusee E, Fawcett R, et al. Thyroid hormone early adjustment in pregnancy (the THERAPY) trial. J Clin Endocrinol Metab 2010;95(7):3234–41.

41. Wilson J, Jungner G. Principles and practice of screening for disease. Geneva (Switzerland): World Health Organization; 1968. p. 34. Public health papers. 2011.

42. Dosiou C, Barnes J, Schwartz A, et al. Cost-effectiveness of universal and risk-based screening for autoimmune thyroid disease in pregnant women. J Clin Endocrinol Metab 2012;97(5):1536–46.

43. De Groot L, Abalovich M, Alexander EK, et al. Management of thyroid dysfunction during pregnancy and postpartum: an endocrine society clinical practice guideline. J Clin Endocrinol Metab 2012;97(8):2543–65.

44. Vaidya B, Anthony S, Bilous M, et al. Detection of thyroid dysfunction in early pregnancy: universal screening or targeted high-risk case finding? J Clin Endocrinol Metab 2007;92(1):203–7.

Thyroid Nodules and Thyroid Cancer in the Pregnant Woman

Trevor E. Angell, MD[a], Erik K. Alexander, MD[b],*

KEYWORDS

- Thyroid nodule • Pregnancy • Thyroid cancer • Fine-needle aspiration • TSH

KEY POINTS

- Thyroid nodules identified during pregnancy should be evaluated with ultrasound and fine-needle aspiration biopsy when indicated to determine the risk of malignancy.
- During gestation, surgery for potential or confirmed low-risk thyroid cancer typically can be delayed until after pregnancy, avoiding maternal risks without increasing adverse cancer outcomes.
- Assessment of thyroid hormone status in women with thyroid nodules is important to optimizing both diagnostic evaluation and maternal thyroid function during gestation.
- Levothyroxine therapy after thyroidectomy needs active management during pregnancy to ensure that increases in dose maintain thyrotropin in the appropriate range.

INTRODUCTION

A thyroid nodule is defined as a discrete lesion within the thyroid gland that can be seen as radiologically distinct from the surrounding thyroid tissue.[1] Thyroid nodules are common in the adult population and are found more frequently in women.[2–5] Although the presence of thyroid nodules increases with age, the burden of disease on young women remains substantial,[6] and the first identification of a thyroid nodule may be during pregnancy. The purpose of thyroid nodule evaluation is to detect possible thyroid cancer and ultimately to guide the ideal management of patients in order to minimize the risks posed by thyroid cancer, thus maximizing health. These principles are perhaps most evident when thyroid nodules or cancer are discovered

Disclosures: Dr T.E. Angell (none). Dr E.K. Alexander, consultant (Veracyte, Inc.).
a Division of Endocrinology and Diabetes, Keck School of Medicine of the University of Southern California, 1333 San Pablo Avenue, BMT-B11, Los Angeles, CA 90033, USA; b The Thyroid Section, Division of Endocrinology, Diabetes, and Hypertension, Brigham & Women's Hospital, Harvard Medical School, 75 Francis Street, Thorn Building 1st Floor, Room 126. Boston, MA 02115, USA
* Corresponding author.
E-mail address: ekalexander@bwh.harvard.edu

in a pregnant woman. The risks and potential contraindications associated with any intervention performed during pregnancy must be taken into account. Pregnancy has a profound influence on thyroid physiology, and thus the impact of gestation on nodule formation, malignant transformation, and cancer behavior must also be considered. This article focuses on the detection, evaluation, and treatment of thyroid nodules and thyroid cancer during pregnancy.

EVALUATION AND MANAGEMENT OF THYROID NODULES DURING PREGNANCY

The estimated prevalence of a palpable thyroid nodule is approximately 5% to 6% in adult women, whereas up to 68% of adults may have a thyroid nodule detectable by imaging, such as computed tomography (CT), magnetic resonance (MR), or ultrasound (US).[2] Although the occurrence of nodules (both solitary and multiple) is more frequent with advancing age, thyroid nodules may be first detected in younger women during pregnancy. Most frequently this is by palpation of the neck and may be influenced by the greater contact with medical care women receive when pregnant. Given the slow rate of thyroid nodule growth,[7,8] most nodules detected during pregnancy were likely present before conception. The average age of pregnancy in the United States has gradually increased over the last 4 decades, and many women now seek pregnancy after 30 years of age.[9] This, combined with the epidemiology and natural history of thyroid nodules, suggests that the frequency of thyroid nodules among women during pregnancy may continue to increase. The ultimate goal of thyroid nodule evaluation is the detection of thyroid cancer, although only 8% to 16% of nodules prove malignant.[2,4,10,11]

The physiologic and hormonal changes that occur in pregnancy seem to affect thyroid nodule formulation and growth. Studies have suggested an association between pregnancy and both the appearance of new nodules and increase in nodule size during gestation.[12,13] Kung and colleagues[12] reported the results of serial US examinations for 221 newly pregnant patients, showing that the proportion of patients with a thyroid nodule increased by nearly 10% from the first to the third trimester. However, most newly detected nodules were very small, measuring less than 5 mm in diameter. Separately, a case-control analysis by Karger and colleagues[13] demonstrated an increased prevalence of nodularity among women previously pregnant in comparison with nulliparous controls. In another study of 26 pregnant women from an iodine-deficiency area, there was an increase in the largest nodule diameter (mean change = 0.7 mm) and a nonsignificant increase in nodule volume during pregnancy, with no increase in nodule formation.[14] It should be emphasized that the clinical impact of such nodule formation may be minimal, and the findings thus far do not indicate a need for routine evaluation for thyroid nodules or serial monitoring of nonmalignant nodules during pregnancy.[15]

The evaluation of a thyroid nodule in a pregnant patient is similar to that of a nonpregnant patient.[9] A thorough medical interview should be performed to identify historical details that increase the risk of thyroid cancer, such as exposure to ionizing radiation in childhood, the presence of thyroid cancer in family members, or high-risk symptoms such as persistent hoarseness of voice, neck pain, or neck lymphadenopathy. The physical examination should define the size, location, and characteristics of a thyroid nodule and findings that raise suspicion for thyroid cancer, including very firm nodules ("rock-hard"), hoarse voice, fixation to surrounding structures, or the presence of lymphadenopathy, particularly when asymmetrically presence on the same side as a thyroid nodule. Following clinical risk assessment, pregnant women with suspected thyroid nodules should undergo US examination and have measurement of serum thyrotropin (thyroid-stimulating hormone [TSH]).

Thyroid US does not use ionizing radiation and is safe during pregnancy. In addition to a description of sizes and locations within the gland of any thyroid nodules identified, the US evaluation should include a sonographic risk assessment. Important features to note are solid versus cystic contents, parenchymal echogenicity (eg, hypo-, iso-, and hyper-echoic), the presence and nature of calcifications (eg, microcalcifications, rim calcifications), nodule margins, and the appearance of abnormal or enlarged regional lymph nodes. Sonographic features most strongly correlated with malignancy are a marked hypoechogenicity, microcalcifications, irregular or invasive margins, and pathologic adenopathy,[16] while other features show less reliability to predict cancer. Assessment of "sonographic patterns" may be useful in stratifying the risk of malignancy,[1,17] but suboptimal reproducibility in the reporting of sonographic features still limits the accuracy of US features and the patterns on which they are based.[18,19]

It is important that all pregnant women with thyroid nodules have an assessment of thyroid function,[15] including the potential use of thyroid hormone supplementation and measurement of serum TSH concentration. Although levothyroxine is the standard recommended form of thyroid hormone supplementation, the inquiry should assure that no other forms of thyroid hormone such as synthetic T3 or natural desiccated preparations are being used. Assessment of TSH serves 2 purposes. First, the presence of a suppressed TSH may suggest an autonomously functioning nodule, potentially modifying the risk of malignancy, but may be difficult to interpret during pregnancy because of physiologic suppression of TSH by human chorionic gonadotropin (hCG) stimulation and the inability to use radioactive iodine assessment. Second, abnormal thyroid findings or use of thyroid hormone supplementation raise the possibility of thyroid dysfunction (especially an underactive thyroid), which is an important concern in pregnancy to identify and manage (discussed later).

Patients with nonsuppressed TSH values should be considered for US-guided fine-needle aspiration biopsy (UG-FNA). This decision should be informed by current clinical guidelines, other literature, and discussion with the patient. In general, solid nodules with sonographic findings classified as moderate to highly suspicious for malignancy should be aspirated when larger than 1 cm.[1] In contrast, nodules without these features, which typically have a low to very low risk of malignancy, should be aspirated when larger than 1.5 to 2.0 cm, respectively.[1] Purely cystic nodules should not be aspirated, as they are benign. Side effects of UG-FNA, beyond mild bruising, are very rare, whereas the information gained from cytologic analysis significantly improves thyroid cancer risk assessment.[1,4,20,21] The Bethesda system for reporting thyroid cytopathology is increasingly used and recommended for cytologic diagnosis of UG-FNA.[1] Conceptually, specimens are categorized as benign if there is an adequate sample in which no features that suggest malignancy are identified. Specimens are classified as malignant if cancer is apparent or as indeterminate when some features of cancer are present without fulfilling sufficient criteria to confirm the diagnosis.[20,21] Approximately 70% of thyroid nodules will be cytologically benign, whereas 5% to 10% will be cytologically malignant and ~5% will be nondiagnostic. However, ~15% to 30% of nodule aspirates are classified as cytologically indeterminate, and the reported frequency of cancer proved by histopathology is broad.[21,22] Performing UG-FNA, including the common practice of using subcutaneous lidocaine, is a safe procedure during pregnancy.[23–26] Pregnancy does not seem to have an effect on the cyologic interpretation or results from thyroid FNA,[27,28] although there are no high-quality prospective data in this regard. As most nodules have been present before (yet detected during) pregnancy, the distribution of FNA cytology results would be expected to mimic that demonstrated for a general nonpregnant population.[4]

The management of thyroid nodules detected during pregnancy should be guided by sonographic and cytologic findings. In general, most cases of thyroid cancer detected during pregnancy behave in an indolent fashion,[13,29] and investigations have failed to show additional harm attributable to the presence of thyroid cancer during pregnancy.[30–33] Therefore, a conservative approach to cytologically indeterminate or malignant nodules is often considered. Moosa and Mazzaferri[30] studied 589 patients with newly diagnosed thyroid cancer, performing a case-control study comparing 61 patients diagnosed during pregnancy with 528 patients diagnosed while not pregnant. The time to treatment was delayed by 15 months in pregnant patients. Despite this delay in treatment, no attributable harm was demonstrated. In a cancer registry study from California, USA, 595 women diagnosed with thyroid cancer during or within 12 months of pregnancy were compared with 2270 age- and sex-matched nonpregnancy thyroid cancer controls without an observed difference in mortality.[31]

More recent studies, however, have stirred controversy regarding the potential for increased aggressiveness of thyroid cancers during pregnancy. Messuti and colleagues[34] noted a high rate of persistent or recurrent disease when thyroid cancer was diagnosed during or shortly following pregnancy. However, serum thyroglobulin levels were commonly greater than 10 ng/mL at the time of radioactive iodine-131 (I^{131}) ablation, raising questions regarding the extent of initial resection and whether this might influence the finding of a biochemically incomplete response. In a separate study by Vannucchi and colleagues,[35] 15 women diagnosed with papillary thyroid carcinoma (PTC) during pregnancy or in the early post-partum period were compared with women with PTC diagnosed greater than 1 year after pregnancy (n = 47) or women with PTC who were nulliparous (n = 61). The percentage of women with persistent disease (defined by the presence after initial surgery and radioactive iodine treatment of metastases to the regional neck lymph node or distant sites, presence of significant thyroglobulin elevation, or persistence of thyroglobulin antibodies for more than 4 years with upward trend) was much higher (60%) in the former group than in the other patients (9.3%). Immunohistochemistry evaluation of tumors in the pregnancy/post-partum group showed a higher proportion expressed estrogen receptor alpha, suggesting a possible mechanism for this phenomenon.[36] In a small prospective clinical study comparing women diagnosed with PTC during or within 12 months of pregnancy with similar nonpregnancy patients,[33] tumors in the group with pregnant women were significantly larger and had a higher percentage of metastatic lymph nodes (mean ± SD 32% ± 29% vs 15% ± 18%, respectively). Pregnant women also had significant more total lymph nodes resected.

Given inconsistent findings between studies and their limitations, these results remain difficult to interpret and do not conclusively indicate greater thyroid cancer risk related to pregnancy. In addition, thyroid surgery during pregnancy does impart higher operative and hospital risks in comparison to nonpregnant patients. Kuy and colleagues[37] investigated 31,356 women undergoing thyroid or parathyroid surgery between the years of 1999 to 2004 and found that in women pregnant at the time of surgery, operative complications (23.9% vs 10.4%), length of stay (2 days vs 1 day), and total cost ($6873 vs $5963) were all increased in comparison to nonpregnant controls. Overall, delay in surgery until after pregnancy seems to be associated with minimal risk and better safety, although further research into outcomes in women with thyroid cancer during pregnancy is warranted.

Thyroid nodules with indeterminate cytology represent a diagnostic dilemma.[1,38] Although diagnostic surgery provides definitive identification of cancer when present, avoiding surgery when possible during pregnancy is preferable. In nonpregnant women, molecular diagnostic testing of cytologically indeterminate thyroid nodules can improve preoperative cancer risk assessment.[39,40] Such tests are not recommended currently in pregnant women, given a lack of data available in this group. Detection of cancer-related genetic mutations or alteration may improve the identification of thyroid cancer. Numerous studies show that a *BRAF* mutation leading to the BRAFV600E-mutated protein guarantees the presence of thyroid cancer and this is unlikely to be effected by pregnancy. Therefore, BRAFV600E testing could be informative, although its frequency is low within indeterminate cytology nodules.[41] BRAFV600E positivity also does not necessarily confirm that the cancer will exhibit aggressive findings that would mandate the urgent intervention of surgery during pregnancy (discussed later). Similarly, the *RET/PTC* fusions are highly specific for thyroid malignancy but occur rarely in samples with indeterminate cytology. Other common gene mutations, particularly in the *RAS* oncogenes (ie, *KRAS*, *NRAS*, and *HRAS*), are less specific for malignancy and are present in nodules with benign behavior.[42,43] Oncogene panels are clinically available via commercial molecular diagnostic tests.[44,45] Gene-expression profiling is a separate method for preoperative risk stratification of indeterminate nodules. Abnormal gene expression reflects altered function of cancer cells, as well as in the tumor microenvironment. A gene expression profiling test is commercially available clinically and has been robustly validated in a nonpregnant population,[46–49] but it is possible that aspects of gene expression are influenced by hormonal changes of pregnancy. Neither form of testing has been prospectively investigated in pregnant women. Because of the paucity of data, the use of molecular testing in pregnant women with indeterminate FNA cytology is not currently recommended.

Indeterminate thyroid nodules are not definitively malignant but when cancerous often represent less aggressive variants of thyroid carcinoma.[50] Harm due to delayed treatment of low-risk, well-differentiated thyroid malignancies in a pregnant patient is rare and must be balanced against the operative risks and complications during pregnancy. The current data provide support for a more conservative approach to pregnant women with thyroid nodules.

EVALUATION AND MANAGEMENT OF THYROID CANCER DURING PREGNANCY

For most patients with possible or confirmed well-differentiated thyroid carcinoma (WDTC) discovered by cytology in early pregnancy, the cancer should be initially assessed and then regularly monitored for evidence of highly aggressive behavior for which intervention during gestation may become necessary.[1] If sonographic evidence of substantial growth, tracheal or vessel invasion, or lymph node involvement is detected, surgery should be considered. If performed, surgery should generally occur in the second trimester before 24 to 26 weeks of gestation. However, most patients will have low-risk WDTC that does not progress significantly during pregnancy. In such cases, surgery can be safely deferred until after delivery. An exception to these recommendations is the rare findings of a more aggressive type of thyroid malignancy (eg, medullary, poorly differentiated, or anaplastic) or clinically aggressive WDTC. In such circumstances, therapy is often warranted during pregnancy, and care must be individualized.

Thyroid tissue growth is stimulated by TSH, and lowering serum TSH reduces the stimulus for cancer growth. If a low-risk cancerous nodule is being followed with a nonoperative approach during pregnancy, targeting a serum TSH level less than 2.0 mU/L can be considered. Levothyroxine initiation, at a starting dose of 50 to 75mcg daily, is generally recommended if TSH concentrations are near-normal but above this goal.[51] Once started, repeat TSH testing is performed after 4 to 5 weeks with continued levothyroxine titration to achieve the TSH goal.

For many nonpregnant patients with WDTC, adjunctive I[131] is administered following surgical resection.[1] I[131] is contraindicated during gestation due to direct radiation-related risk of teratogenicity as well as because maternally administered I[131] readily crosses the placenta and may damage or destroy the fetal thyroid tissue by the second trimester. If radioactive iodine therapy is indicated, this must be delayed until the postpartum period and ideally until after cessation of lactation because of the concentration of I[131] is breast milk. Women who have surgery for WDTC during pregnancy should be followed-up conservatively with regular monitoring and TSH suppressive therapy.

MANAGEMENT OF PREEXISTING THYROID CANCER DURING PREGNANCY

Women with preexisting thyroid carcinoma will continue to require monitoring and management during any new pregnancy. Serum thyroglobulin (Tg) is usually the most sensitive marker for detecting recurrent or residual disease. In patients who have not undergone I[131] ablation, precise cut-offs indicating the presence or absence of thyroid cancer are less certain, but a maternal serum Tg concentration less than 2 ng/dL supports the absence of active thyroid malignancy. In contrast, Tg greater than or equal to 2IU/L or increasing concentrations over time[1,52] suggest recurrence or progression of disease. Approximately 20% of patients with thyroid cancer harbor antibodies to Tg (TgAb), which are not pathogenic, but may interfere with Tg measurement.[53] For the most common assay methods used for Tg, the presence of TgAb may lead to falsely low or undetected Tg values.[54,55] Initial screening for TgAb should be performed before serum Tg measurement and is performed by most laboratories if Tg assessment is requested. If TgAb are detected, the test for Tg may be canceled or assessed by a different method to avoid interference, but all Tg results obtained in the presence of TgAb require cautious interpretation. The persistent presence of TgAb, and particularly increasing levels over time, are themselves a signal of concern for potential persistent thyroid cancer.[1,56]

For patients in whom Tg or TgAb suggest persistent thyroid cancer, a thorough physical examination and neck US should be performed to identify an anatomic source. The use of additional imaging modalities, such as CT, PET, or MRI, to search for metastatic disease is complicated by contraindications that exist during pregnancy, and the need for such testing should be individualized based on the likelihood of detecting disease that would be treated during pregnancy balanced against the risks of testing.

Thyroid hormone management in women who have undergone thyroidectomy is essential both to achieve adequate TSH suppression as a cornerstone of differentiated thyroid cancer management and to anticipate the changes in thyroid hormone physiology that occur during pregnancy.[1,15] Pregnancy is a period of increased thyroid hormone need representing a physiologic thyroidal "stress test." The reasons for this include increased iodine excretion, greater serum binding of thyroid hormone to circulating thyroxine binding globulin, and stimulation of the TSH receptor by increasing concentrations of hCG.[15,57] Indeed, thyroid hormone production increases by an average of 40% during gestation.[58] In patients with impaired thyroid function (whether or not requiring levothyroxine therapy prepregnancy), or in whom the thyroid gland has been removed surgically, this stimulated increase in thyroxine production cannot occur endogenously and the increasing demand of thyroxine during gestation will induce maternal hypothyroidism. In such cases, initiation or elevation of levothyroxine are necessary to ensure an appropriate serum TSH concentration. The pattern of increasing demand during gestation has been carefully studied and begins very early in gestation.[58] Demand thereafter increases linearly through approximately 16 to

20 weeks of gestation, where the maximal requirement is often identified. After midgestation, the increased requirement for thyroxine plateaus but is sustained. On delivery, thyroxine requirements return to pregestational levels.

In a pregnant woman evaluated for a thyroid nodule or new thyroid cancer, thyroid function assessment should be performed, and if thyroid dysfunction is identified (or if thyroid removal is impending) levothyroxine is given with the goal of maintaining normal thyroid function. If this occurs in the first half of pregnancy, maternal serum TSH should be assessed every 3 to 4 weeks thereafter until the 20th week of gestation. If levothyroxine is started after the 20th week, thyroid hormone levels are more stable and TSH reassessment should occur roughly 4 weeks after each new dose until TSH goal is achieved.

The goal TSH level to which levothyroxine dosing should be titrated during pregnancy will depend on the patient's diagnosis. For women with a diagnosis of thyroid cancer, before or during the pregnancy, the TSH goal should reflect the goal for TSH suppression that would otherwise be recommended for the management of the malignant disease.[1] Although the TSH suppression goal varies based on the degree of risk for persistent disease, even mild suppression (0.5–2.0 mIU/L) recommended for low-risk thyroid cancers provides sufficient thyroid hormone believed to minimize the risk of adverse pregnancy outcomes.[15] For pregnant women without thyroid cancer, but who had previous thyroid surgery or abnormal thyroid function during evaluation, recommendations are more complex. For women taking levothyroxine, the dose should be adjusted, with the goal of maintaining a serum TSH concentration less than 2.5 mIU/L in the first trimester.[15] In women who are newly pregnant, this can be achieved by adding an additional 2 pills per week and performing repeat TSH assessments every 4 weeks to assure goal TSH is maintained.[59] Alternative dosing schemes have been developed, although there is currently no clear evidence supporting one versus another regimen.[60] For previously euthyroid women not taking levothyroxine, those with overt hypothyroidism or TSH concentration greater than 10 mIU/L should receive levothyroxine treatment. Although the ideal TSH and thyroxine concentrations during pregnancy are still a matter of considerable debate and study, the presence of thyroperoxidase antibody (TPOAb) seems to modify the risk of adverse pregnancy outcomes, and levothyroxine initiation for TPOAb-positive women when TSH is greater than 2.5 mIU/L in the first trimester is recommended.[15,61]

In conclusion, the identification of thyroid nodules occurs frequently during pregnancy. US and UG-FNA can be safely performed during pregnancy and provide important information regarding overall cancer risk assessment. The approach to thyroid surgery during pregnancy is generally conservative. Most thyroid cancers detected during pregnancy will not pose risk to the patient or fetus during gestation. Therefore, the decision to pursue thyroidectomy must be individualized, weighing the risks and benefits of any intervention against those of conservative monitoring. In rare circumstances, high-risk scenarios necessitate thyroidectomy during pregnancy. Maternal serum TSH concentrations should be regularly assessed during the first half of pregnancy, to assure sufficient levels. Through a balanced and informed approach to the clinical care of this unique population, outcomes can be optimized for both the pregnant mother and the developing fetus.

REFERENCES

1. Haugen BR, Alexander EK, Bible KC, et al. 2015 American Thyroid Association Management guidelines for adult patients with thyroid nodules and differentiated thyroid cancer: the American Thyroid Association guidelines task force on thyroid nodules and differentiated thyroid cancer. Thyroid 2016;26:1–133.

2. Burman KD, Wartofsky L. Clinical practice. Thyroid nodules. N Engl J Med 2015; 373:2347–56.

3. Frates MC, Benson CB, Doubilet PM, et al. Prevalence and distribution of carcinoma in patients with solitary and multiple thyroid nodules on sonography. J Clin Endocrinol Metab 2006;91:3411–7.

4. Yassa L, Cibas ES, Benson CB, et al. Long-term assessment of a multidisciplinary approach to thyroid nodule diagnostic evaluation. Cancer Cytopathol 2007;111: 508–16.

5. Guth S, Theune U, Aberle J, et al. Very high prevalence of thyroid nodules detected by high frequency (13 MHz) ultrasound examination. Eur J Clin Invest 2009;39:699–706.

6. Kwong N, Medici M, Angell TE, et al. The influence of patient age on thyroid nodule formation, multinodularity, and thyroid cancer risk. J Clin Endocrinol Metab 2015;100:4434–40.

7. Durante C, Costante G, Lucisano G, et al. The natural history of benign thyroid nodules. JAMA 2015;313:926–35.

8. Angell TE, Vyas CM, Medici M, et al. Differential growth rates of benign vs. malignant thyroid nodules. J Clin Endocrinol Metab 2017;102:4642–7.

9. Martin JA, Hamilton BE, Osterman MJK, et al. National vital statistics report. 2015. Available at: http://www.cdc.gov/nchs/data/nvsr/nvsr64/nvsr64_01.pdf. Accessed May 30, 2019.

10. Siegel RL, Miller KD, Jemal A. Cancer statistics, 2018. CA Cancer J Clin 2018; 68:7–30.

11. Brito JP, Morris JC, Montori VM. Thyroid cancer: zealous imaging has increased detection and treatment of low risk tumours. BMJ 2013;347:f4706.

12. Kung AW, Chau MT, Lao TT, et al. The effect of pregnancy on thyroid nodule formation. J Clin Endocrinol Metab 2002;87:1010–4.

13. Karger S, Schötz S, Stumvoll M, et al. Impact of pregnancy on prevalence of goitre and nodular thyroid disease in women living in a region of borderline sufficient iodine supply. Horm Metab Res 2010;42:137–42.

14. Sahin SB, Ogullar S, Ural UM, et al. Alterations of thyroid volume and nodular size during and after pregnancy in a severe iodine-deficient area. Clin Endocrinol (Oxf) 2014;81:762–8.

15. Alexander EK, Pearce EN, Brent GA, et al. 2017 guidelines of the American Thyroid Association for the diagnosis and management of thyroid disease during pregnancy and the postpartum. Thyroid 2017;27:315–89.

16. Moon HJ, Sung JM, Kim EK, et al. Diagnostic performance of gray-scale US and elastography in solid thyroid nodules. Radiology 2012;262:1002–13.

17. Grant EG, Tessler FN, Hoang JK, et al. Thyroid ultrasound reporting lexicon: white paper of the ACR thyroid imaging, reporting and data system (TIRADS) committee. J Am Coll Radiol 2015;12:1272–9.

18. Hoang JK, Middleton WD, Farjat AE, et al. Interobserver variability of sonographic features used in the American College of Radiology Thyroid Imaging Reporting and Data System. AJR Am J Roentgenol 2018;211:162–7.

19. Grani G, Lamartina L, Cantisani V, et al. Interobserver agreement of various thyroid imaging reporting and data systems. Endocr Connect 2018;7:1–7.

20. Cibas ES, Ali SZ. The Bethesda system for reporting thyroid cytopathology. Thyroid 2009;19:1159–65.

21. Bongiovanni M, Crippa S, Baloch Z, et al. Comparison of 5-tiered and 6-tiered diagnostic systems for the reporting of thyroid cytopathology: a multi-institutional study. Cancer Cytopathol 2012;120:117–25.

22. Cibas ES, Ali SZ. The 2017 Bethesda system for reporting thyroid cytopathology. Thyroid 2017;27:1341–6.
23. Belfiore A, La Rosa GL. Fine-needle aspiration biopsy of the thyroid. Endocrinol Metab Clin North Am 2001;30:361–400.
24. Goellner JR, Gharib H, Grant CS, et al. Fine needle aspiration cytology of the thyroid, 1980 to 1986. Acta Cytol 1987;31:587–90.
25. Choe W, McDougall IR. Thyroid cancer in pregnant women: diagnostic and therapeutic management. Thyroid 1994;4:433–5.
26. Hamburger JI. Thyroid nodules in pregnancy. Thyroid 1992;2:165–8.
27. Tan GH, Gharib H, Goellner JR, et al. Management of thyroid nodules in pregnancy. Arch Intern Med 1996;156:2317–20.
28. Marley EF, Oertel YC. Fine-needle aspiration of thyroid lesions in 57 pregnant and postpartum women. Diagn Cytopathol 1997;16:122–5.
29. Rosen IB, Korman M, Walfish PG. Thyroid nodular disease in pregnancy: current diagnosis and management. Clin Obstet Gynecol 1997;40:81–9.
30. Moosa M, Mazzaferri EL. Outcome of differentiated thyroid cancer diagnosed in pregnant women. J Clin Endocrinol Metab 1997;82:2862–6.
31. Yasmeen S, Cress R, Romano PS, et al. Thyroid cancer in pregnancy. Int J Gynaecol Obstet 2005;91:15–20.
32. Herzon FS, Morris DM, Segal MN, et al. Coexistent thyroid cancer and pregnancy. Arch Otolaryngol Head Neck Surg 1994;120:1191–3.
33. Lee JC, Zhao JT, Clifton-Bligh RJ, et al. Papillary thyroid carcinoma in pregnancy: a variant of the disease? Ann Surg Oncol 2012;19:4210–6.
34. Messuti I, Corvisieri S, Bardesono F, et al. Impact of pregnancy on prognosis of differentiated thyroid cancer: clinical and molecular features. Eur J Endocrinol 2014;170:659–66.
35. Vannucchi G, Perrino M, Rossi S, et al. Clinical and molecular features of differentiated thyroid cancer diagnosed during pregnancy. Eur J Endocrinol 2010; 162:145–51.
36. Vannucchi G, De Leo S, Perrino M, et al. Impact of estrogen and progesterone receptor expression on the clinical and molecular features of papillary thyroid cancer. Eur J Endocrinol 2015;173:29–36.
37. Kuy S, Roman SA, Desai R, et al. Outcomes following thyroid and parathyroid surgery in pregnant women. Arch Surg 2009;144:399–406.
38. Durante C, Grani G, Lamartina L, et al. The diagnosis and management of thyroid nodules: a review. JAMA 2018;319:914–24.
39. Beaudenon-Huibregtse S, Alexander EK, Guttler RB, et al. Centralized molecular testing for oncogenic gene mutations complements the local cytopathologic diagnosis of thyroid nodules. Thyroid 2014;10:1479–87.
40. Nikiforov YE, Ohori NP, Hodak SP, et al. Impact of mutational testing on the diagnosis and management of patients with cytologically indeterminate thyroid nodules: a prospective analysis of 1056 FNA samples. J Clin Endocrinol Metab 2011;96:3390–7.
41. Kleiman DA, Sporn MJ, Beninato T, et al. Preoperative BRAF(V600E) mutation screening is unlikely to alter initial surgical treatment of patients with indeterminate thyroid nodules: a prospective case series of 960 patients. Cancer 2013; 119:1495–502.
42. Angell TE. RAS-positive thyroid nodules. Curr Opin Endocrinol Diabetes Obes 2017;24:372–6.
43. Medici M, Kwong N, Angell TE, et al. The variable phenotype and low-risk nature of RAS-positive thyroid nodules. BMC Med 2015;13:184–9.

44. Steward DL, Carty SE, Sippel RS, et al. Performance of a multigene genomic classifier in thyroid nodules with indeterminate cytology: a prospective blinded multicenter study. JAMA Oncol 2018. https://doi.org/10.1001/jamaoncol.2018. 4616.

45. Labourier E, Shifrin A, Busseniers AE, et al. Molecular testing for miRNA, mRNA, and DNA on fine-needle aspiration improves the preoperative diagnosis of thyroid nodules with indeterminate cytology. J Clin Endocrinol Metab 2015;100: 2743–50.

46. Alexander EK, Kennedy GC, Baloch ZW, et al. Preoperative diagnosis of benign thyroid nodules with indeterminate cytology. N Engl J Med 2012;367:705–15.

47. Patel KN, Angell TE, Babiarz J, et al. Performance of a genomic sequencing classifier for the preoperative diagnosis of cytologically indeterminate thyroid nodules. JAMA Surg 2018;153:817–24.

48. Alexander EK, Schorr M, Klopper J, et al. Multicenter clinical experience with the Afirma gene expression classifier. J Clin Endocrinol Metab 2014;99:119–25.

49. Roth MY, Witt RL, Steward DL. Molecular testing for thyroid nodules: review and current state. Cancer 2018;124:888–98.

50. Liu X, Medici M, Kwong N, et al. Bethesda categorization of thyroid nodule cytology and prediction of thyroid cancer type and prognosis. Thyroid 2016;26: 256–61.

51. McLeod DS, Watters KF, Carpenter AD, et al. Thyrotropin and thyroid cancer diagnosis: a systematic review and dose-response meta-analysis. J Clin Endocrinol Metab 2012;97:2682–92.

52. Webb RC, Howard RS, Stojadinovic A, et al. The utility of serum thyroglobulin measurement at the time of remnant ablation for predicting disease-free status in patients with differentiated thyroid cancer: a meta-analysis involving 3947 patients. J Clin Endocrinol Metab 2012;97:2754–63.

53. Latrofa F, Ricci D, Montanelli L, et al. Lymphocytic thyroiditis on histology correlates with serum thyroglobulin autoantibodies in patients with papillary thyroid carcinoma: impact on detection of serum thyroglobulin. J Clin Endocrinol Metab 2012;97:2380–7.

54. Spencer CA, Takeuchi M, Kazarosyan M, et al. Serum thyroglobulin autoantibodies: prevalence, influence on serum thyroglobulin measurement, and prognostic significance in patients with differentiated thyroid carcinoma. J Clin Endocrinol Metab 1998;83:1121–7.

55. Netzel BC, Grebe SK, Carranza Leon BG, et al. Thyroglobulin (Tg) testing revisited: Tg assays, TgAb assays, and correlation of results with clinical outcomes. J Clin Endocrinol Metab 2015;100:E1074–83.

56. Matrone A, Latrofa F, Torregrossa L, et al. Changing trend of thyroglobulin antibodies in patients with differentiated thyroid cancer treated with total thyroidectomy without 131I ablation. Thyroid 2018;28:871–9.

57. Korevaar TIM, Medici M, Visser TJ, et al. Thyroid disease in pregnancy: new insights in diagnosis and clinical management. Nat Rev Endocrinol 2017;13: 610–22.

58. Alexander EK, Marqusee E, Lawrence J, et al. Timing and magnitude of increases in levothyroxine requirements during pregnancy in women with hypothyroidism. N Engl J Med 2004;351:25–33.

59. Yassa L, Marqusee E, Fawcett R, et al. Thyroid hormone early adjustment in pregnancy (the THERAPY) trial. J Clin Endocrinol Metab 2010;95:3234–41.

60. Sullivan SD, Downs E, Popoveniuc G, et al. Randomized trial comparing two algorithms for levothyroxine dose adjustment in pregnant women with primary hypothyroidism. J Clin Endocrinol Metab 2017;102:3499–507.
61. Nazarpour S, Ramezani Tehrani F, Simbar M, et al. Effects of levothyroxine treatment on pregnancy outcomes in pregnant women with autoimmune thyroid disease. Eur J Endocrinol 2017;176:253–65.

Pituitary Tumors in Pregnancy

Wenyu Huang, MD, PhD, Mark E. Molitch, MD*

KEYWORDS

- Pituitary tumor • Pregnancy • Prolactinoma • Acromegaly • Cushing disease

KEY POINTS

- About 18% of prolactin-secreting macroadenomas enlarge significantly during pregnancy, compared with 2.5% of prolactin-secreting microadenomas.
- In women with prolactinomas, dopamine agonists should be discontinued on confirmation of pregnancy.
- Dopamine agonists can be used to treat symptomatic enlargement of prolactinomas during pregnancy.
- In patients with acromegaly, the risks of gestational diabetes and hypertension are increased. Treatment of the acromegaly is usually not needed during pregnancy.
- In patients with Cushing disease found in pregnancy, the treatment of choice is surgery in the second trimester.

INTRODUCTION

Pituitary adenomas can affect fertility and pregnancy outcomes, if pregnancy does ensue, because of oversecretion of hormones as well as by causing hypopituitarism. In addition, the pregnancy itself alters hormone secretion and pituitary tumor size, complicating the evaluation and management of patients with pituitary neoplasms. The influence of various types of therapy on the developing fetus also affects therapeutic decision making.

PROLACTINOMA AND PREGNANCY

Hyperprolactinemia is a common cause of female infertility.[1] When women with prolactinomas get pregnant, 2 important issues arise: (1) the effects of the dopamine agonist on early fetal development; and (2) the effect of pregnancy on prolactinoma size.[2]

Disclosure: The authors have nothing to disclose related to this article.
Division of Endocrinology, Metabolism and Molecular Medicine, Northwestern University Feinberg School of Medicine, 645 North Michigan Avenue, Suite 530, Chicago, IL 60611, USA
* Corresponding author.
E-mail address: molitch@northwestern.edu

Endocrinol Metab Clin N Am 48 (2019) 569–581
https://doi.org/10.1016/j.ecl.2019.05.004

Effects of Dopamine Agonists on the Developing Fetus

For patients with prolactinomas, dopamine agonists are the treatment of choice, because they are effective in correcting the hyperprolactinemia and restoring ovulation in more than 90% of women.[3–5] In general, dopamine agonists should be stopped on confirmation of pregnancy. Bromocriptine has been shown to cross the placenta in human studies[1]; cabergoline has been shown to do so in animal studies but such data are lacking in humans.

In more than 6000 pregnancies, bromocriptine has not been associated with adverse pregnancy outcomes (**Table 1**).[1,2] Bromocriptine has been used throughout gestation in more than 100 women, with no abnormalities noted in the infants except for 1 with an undescended testicle and another with a talipes deformity.[1,2]

Data regarding exposure to cabergoline in pregnancy have been reported in more than 1000 cases (see **Table 1**). There is no increase in malformations or other adverse pregnancy outcomes,[1,2,6–8] including up to 12 years' follow-up after exposure[6,8,9] (see **Table 1**). A summary of cabergoline use throughout gestation indicated that healthy infants were delivered at term in 13 and at 36 weeks in 1, but 1 had an intrauterine death at 34 weeks when the mother had severe preeclampsia.[7,10]

In a review of 176 pregnancies, quinagolide (not available in the United States) was associated with 24 spontaneous abortions, 1 ectopic pregnancy, 1 stillbirth at 31 weeks of gestation, and 9 fetal malformations.[11] Thus, quinagolide does not seem to be safe for pregnancy.

Table 1
Pregnancy outcomes for women who became pregnant while taking bromocriptine or cabergoline, compared with what is expected in the normal population

	Bromocriptine (N)	Bromocriptine (%)	Cabergoline (N)	Cabergoline (%)	Normal (%)
Pregnancies	6272	100	1061	100	100
Spontaneous abortions	620	9.9	77	7.6	10–15
Terminations	75	1.2	66[a]	6.5	20
Ectopic	31	0.5	3	0.3	1.0–1.5
Hydatidiform moles	11	0.2	1	0.1	0.1–0.15
Deliveries (known duration)	4139	100	791	100	100
At term (>37 wk)	3620	87.5	715[b]	90.4	87.3
Preterm (<37 wk)	519	12.5	76	9.6	12.7
Deliveries (known outcome)	5120	100	670	100	100
Single births	5031	98.3	655	97.8	96.8
Multiple births	89	1.7	15	2.2	3.2
Babies (known details)	5246	100	908	100	100
Normal	5061	98.2	884	97.4	97
With malformations	95	1.8	24	2.6	3.0

[a] Fourteen of these terminations were for malformations.
[b] Seven of these births were stillbirths.
Data from Refs.[1,2,7,15]

In contrast with the earlier reassuring information regarding cabergoline and bromocriptine, Hurault-Delarue and colleagues[12] reported some adverse outcomes of dopamine agonist use. Of the 57,408 mother-baby outcome pairs, 183 (0.3%) had received dopamine agonists at some time during their pregnancies (75% in the first trimester).[12] Compared with a control group, dopamine agonist exposure was associated with an increased risk of preterm birth and early pregnancy loss and an insignificant increase in fetal malformations but no difference in psychomotor development at ages 9 and 24 months.[12] There were no differences between the dopamine agonists with respect to these outcomes.

Effect of Pregnancy on Prolactinoma Size

The increasing level of estrogen stimulates lactotroph hyperplasia and an increase in prolactin (PRL) levels over the course of pregnancy.[13] In normal pregnancy, MRI scans show a gradual increase in pituitary volume to a final height of 12 mm.[14]

Prolactinomas can enlarge during pregnancy because of high estrogen levels and/or the discontinuation of the dopamine agonist (**Table 2**). The risk of symptomatic (headaches, visual field defects) tumor enlargement in pregnant women with microprolactinomas is 2.5%, 18.1% for macroprolactinomas with no prior surgery or irradiation, and 4.7% for macroadenomas with prior surgery/irradiation.[1,2,15] In a small proportion of those cases, the tumor enlargement reflected tumor apoplexy[16]; however, the true incidence of apoplexy is unknown. In most cases with tumor enlargement, reintroduction of the dopamine agonist was successful in reversing the problem and surgery was rarely required.

Postpartum PRL levels and tumor sizes often decrease compared with values before pregnancy,[1,2,17] but this has not been observed in all series.[18] Women with prolactinomas can breastfeed. Reinstitution of dopamine agonist has to await the cessation of breastfeeding and is done only in women who remain anovulatory.

Management of Prolactinoma During Pregnancy

Dopamine agonists seem to be the best primary treatment because of their efficacy in restoring ovulation and very low (2.5%) risk of clinically serious tumor enlargement. Compared with bromocriptine, cabergoline is better tolerated, more efficacious, and is similarly safe. Transsphenoidal surgery causes a permanent reduction of PRL levels in only 60% to 70% of cases and entails morbidity and mortality, albeit at low rates.[4,19] Pregnancy can generally be achieved in more than 85% of patients with dopamine agonists or surgery.[8,18,20] Radiotherapy is not warranted for patients with microadenomas because of the risk of long-term sequelae, especially hypopituitarism.[21]

Patients with a microadenoma or a small intrasellar macroadenoma who were treated with a dopamine agonist and had medication withdrawal after conception need only to be followed clinically throughout gestation. PRL levels do not always increase during pregnancy in women with prolactinomas, even in those with tumor enlargement and PRL levels may rise significantly without any tumor size increase.[22] Therefore, periodic checking of PRL levels is not recommended.[5] Because of the low incidence of tumor enlargement, visual field testing and MRI scanning are only performed in patients who become symptomatic. Karaca and colleagues[7] showed MRI confirmed tumor enlargement only in 4 out of 10 patients suspected clinically to have tumor enlargement. There are no data documenting harm to the developing fetus from MRI scans.[23] Recently, slight increases in risks of stillbirths, neonatal deaths, and the broad outcome of any rheumatological, inflammatory, or infiltrative skin condition were shown with first-trimester gadolinium exposure.[24] No adverse effects from MRI

Table 2
Enlargement of prolactinomas during pregnancy

Series, Year	Microadenomas			Macroadenomas No Prior Treatment			Macroadenomas Prior Treatment		
	Total (N)	Enlarged (N)	Enlarged (%)	Total (N)	Enlarged (N)	Enlarged (%)	Total (N)	Enlarged (N)	Enlarged (%)
Gemzell & Wang,[73] 1979	85	5		46	20		70	5	
Molitch,[20] 1985	246	4		45	7		46	2	
Holmgren et al,[74] 1986	26	3		4	2		5	0	
Ampudia et al,[75] 1992	8	1		1	0		4	0	
Kupersmith et al,[48] 1994	54	0		4	4		0	0	
Rossi et al,[76] 1995	22	2		3	1		2	0	
Badawy et al,[77] 1997	16	0		0	0		0	0	
Mallmann et al,[78] 2002	5	0		3	1		0	0	
Bronstein et al,[79] 2002	48	1		30	11		21	0	
Ono et al,[8] 2010	56	0		29	0		0	0	
Lebbe et al,[9] 2010	45	2		15	3		0	0	
Stalldecker et al,[6] 2010	47	0		34	0		0	0	
Auriemma et al,[80] 2013	76	0		10	0		0	0	
Domingue et al,[17] 2014a	30	0		14	1		0	0	
Rastogi et al,[15] 2016	0	0		33	0		0	0	
Karaca et al,[7] 2018	36	2		17	2		0	0	
Total	800	20	2.5	288	52	18.1	148	7	4.7

a Analysis of tumor growth from this series: personal communication from D. Maiter, 2015.

with or without gadolinium have been shown in the late second or third trimesters. In clinical practice, it is important to document a significant increase in tumor size before instituting an intervention, such as restarting a dopamine agonist or surgery. If the headache is sudden, it may be caused by pituitary apoplexy, which may require hormone replacement if there is sudden onset of hypopituitarism.[16]

In patients with a larger macroadenoma, it is helpful to have a baseline MRI scan just before pregnancy. There is no best therapeutic approach in such patients. The most common approach is to stop the dopamine agonist after pregnancy is diagnosed. If there was substantial shrinkage of a very large tumor with the dopamine agonist, then stopping the drug abruptly might cause a sudden enlargement of the tumor. In such a case, the wisest course could be to continue the dopamine agonist. Another approach is to debulk the tumor via transsphenoidal surgery, which reduces the risk of serious tumor enlargement, but cases of tumor expansion during pregnancy after such surgery have been reported.[25] After surgical debulking, a dopamine agonist is generally required to normalize PRL levels and allow ovulation. A third approach is to give the dopamine agonist continuously throughout gestation, but data regarding effects on the fetus are meager; therefore, such treatment cannot be recommended without reservation. In contrast, should pregnancy at an advanced stage be discovered in a woman taking bromocriptine or cabergoline, the data are reassuring and do not justify therapeutic abortion.

For patients with macroadenomas treated with a dopamine agonist alone or after surgery, careful follow-up with monthly to 3-monthly formal visual field testing is warranted. Repeat MRI scanning is reserved for patients with symptoms of tumor enlargement and/or visual field defect.

Should symptomatic tumor enlargement occur with any of these approaches, reinstitution of the dopamine agonist is probably less harmful to the mother and child than surgery. Any type of surgery during pregnancy results in a 1.5-fold and 5-fold increase in fetal loss in the first and second trimester respectively, but without risk of congenital malformations.[25,26] In addition, pregnant women have significantly increased risks of postoperative complications, including infections and even mortality.[27] However, such medical therapy must be very closely monitored, and transsphenoidal surgery or delivery (if the pregnancy is far enough advanced) should be performed if there is no response to the dopamine agonist and vision is progressively worsening.

Although suckling stimulates PRL secretion in normal women for the first few weeks to months postpartum, there are no data to suggest that breastfeeding can cause tumor growth. Thus, there seems to be no reason to discourage nursing in women with prolactinomas.

CUSHING DISEASE AND PREGNANCY
Changes of Hypothalamic-Pituitary-Adrenal Axis During Pregnancy

Normal pregnancy is associated with profound changes of the hypothalamic-pituitary-adrenal (HPA) axis, including a 2-fold to 4-fold increase in serum total and free cortisol and urine free cortisol (UFC) levels, preserved but blunted circadian rhythm of cortisol, enhanced response of cortisol to adrenocorticotropic hormone (ACTH), increased corticotropin-releasing hormone (CRH) and ACTH levels, and desensitization of CRH and ACTH secretion to the negative feedback of cortisol.[28]

Cushing Disease in Pregnancy

Cushing syndrome is very rare in pregnancy. Cushing disease accounts for 30% to 40% of Cushing syndrome during pregnancy, in contrast with 70% in the general population.[28] Adrenal causes of Cushing syndrome, mostly adenoma and hyperplasia but even carcinoma, make up about 50% of the cases of Cushing syndrome first found in pregnancy.[29]

Effect of Cushing Disease on Pregnancy

Untreated Cushing syndrome exerts a significant deleterious impact on pregnancy outcomes. Maternal morbidities caused by hypercortisolism occur in 70% of cases and include hypertension, preeclampsia, eclampsia, diabetes, and hyperlipidemia.[29] Other complications include osteoporosis, fracture, impaired wound healing, and psychiatric disorders.[28] However, maternal mortality is rare. Fetal complications from Cushing syndrome during gestation include early spontaneous abortion, prematurity, and intrauterine growth restriction,[30] with fetal mortality occurring in up to 20% of cases.[28]

Diagnosis of Cushing Disease During Pregnancy

The complex changes of the HPA axis during pregnancy make the diagnosis of Cushing disease a major challenge. Many of the abnormalities of the HPA axis found in nongravid patients with Cushing syndrome can be seen in normal pregnancy, including increased cortisol levels, reduced inhibition of the HPA axis by exogenous glucocorticoid, and a blunted circadian rhythm of cortisol. In addition, the symptoms and signs of Cushing syndrome also overlap with those seen in normal pregnancy; for example, weight gain, mood changes, and fatigue.[31]

Even though 24-hour UFC level increases during pregnancy, a level higher than 3-fold of the upper limit of normal has been proposed to suggest Cushing syndrome during pregnancy.[28,31] Late-night salivary cortisol levels also undergo a gradual increase during normal pregnancy. However, using the cutoff values of 0.255 μg/dL (7.0 nmol/L), 0.260 μg/dL (7.2 nmol/L), and 0.285 μg/dL (7.9 nmol/L) for first, second, and third trimesters respectively yields high sensitivity (>80%) and specificity (>90%) in separating Cushing disease from normal gestational changes.[32] The 1-mg dexamethasone overnight suppression test is not reliable for the diagnosis of Cushing syndrome, because more than 60% of normal pregnant women may have abnormal cortisol levels after dexamethasone.[28]

The differential diagnosis of ACTH-independent and ACTH-dependent Cushing syndrome can usually start with an ACTH level, adrenal ultrasonography, and 8-mg dexamethasone suppression test. Importantly, up to 50% of women with adrenal Cushing syndrome may have nonsuppressed ACTH levels during pregnancy caused by placental CRH stimulation and ACTH production.[28] A borderline low or suppressed ACTH level, no response to the suppression by 8-mg dexamethasone, and an adrenal mass on the ultrasonography scan all suggest ACTH-independent Cushing syndrome.[28] When adrenal ultrasonography identifies an adrenal lesion, noncontrast MRI can be used to further characterize the lesion. In patients suspected to have Cushing disease, in addition to the suppressed cortisol level by 8-mg dexamethasone, an increase in ACTH after CRH injection usually suggests Cushing disease. Cushing syndrome caused by ectopic ACTH or with an adrenal cause usually fails to response to exogenous dexamethasone and CRH. Pituitary MRI without contrast is necessary to evaluate pituitary lesions during pregnancy but many patients with Cushing disease have very small microadenomas.[28,31] Because of concern for radiation exposure, inferior petrosal sinus sampling should be reserved for the patients who are difficult to diagnose even after the noninvasive tests.[28]

Management of Cushing Disease During Pregnancy

Reported treatments of Cushing disease during pregnancy include watchful monitoring, surgery, and medication. In a review of 181 pregnancies, Caimari and colleagues[33] found that successful treatment during pregnancy resulted in improved outcomes of low birth weight and preterm birth. For patients with mild disease, it may be reasonable to wait until delivery to treat Cushing disease.[34] However, comorbidities should be adequately controlled during pregnancy.

For patients requiring treatment during pregnancy, transsphenoidal surgery in the second trimester seems to be the treatment of choice.[31] Bilateral adrenalectomy can be considered in those in whom transsphenoidal surgery and medical treatment are not feasible and the patient needs rapid resolution of the hypercortisolism.[31] After either pituitary or adrenal surgery, patients may develop adrenal insufficiency and replacement with hydrocortisone and mineralocorticoid (only after adrenal surgery) are required.

If a patient is not eligible for or refuses surgery, or has failure of surgery, then medical treatments can be considered for those with severe Cushing disease in order to achieve improvement of symptoms, control of tumor or complications, and to improve fetal outcomes. Cabergoline has been used in uncontrolled Cushing disease during pregnancy and seems to confer good control of the disease.[35,36] Ketoconazole inhibits steroidogenesis and seemed to be safe and not associated with congenital malformation, including sexual development.[35,37] Metyrapone crosses the placenta and has the potential of affecting fetal steroidogenesis.[31] Its use during the second and third trimesters was not associated with fetal complications.[37] However, because of the accumulation of deoxycorticosterone caused by metyrapone, maternal hypertension and preeclampsia may be exacerbated.[38] Pasireotide is a somatostatin analogue (SSA) and is approved to treat Cushing disease, but its use in pregnancy has not been reported.[21,39] Although mifepristone can be used to treat Cushing syndrome,[40] it is contraindicated during pregnancy given its antagonism of progesterone receptor.

ACROMEGALY AND PREGNANCY

Changes in Growth Hormone, Growth Hormone Variant, and Insulin-like Growth Factor 1 During Normal Pregnancy and Pregnancy Complicated by Acromegaly

Placenta-derived growth hormone (GH) variant starts to appear in maternal circulation around gestational week 15 to 17 and is released in a continuous manner. It increases throughout pregnancy and becomes the predominant circulating form of GH in the second half of pregnancy. The placental GH-variant stimulates insulin-like growth factor 1 (IGF-1) production.[41] In contrast, pituitary GH declines to very low levels in the later part of pregnancy, presumably because of negative feedback of increasing levels of IGF-1.[38,42]

Compared with the decline of pituitary GH in normal pregnancy, autonomous GH secretion from a pituitary adenoma in acromegaly is not suppressed by the increasing IGF-1 level. However, placental GH-variant secretion is similar in both acromegalic and normal pregnancies. Therefore, pituitary GH and placental GH variant are both present at high concentrations in maternal circulation in late gestation.[38] Interestingly, IGF-1 levels in acromegalic patients may decrease during early pregnancy, even in those without medical treatment.[43]

Interaction Between Pregnancy and Acromegaly

Complications associated with acromegaly, including hypertension, hyperglycemia, and cardiac disease, potentially could worsen during pregnancy.[38,43–45] However, such exacerbations are rare.[43,44] Tumor enlargement in patients with acromegaly is uncommon, with only 5 cases reported.[7,46–49] Most studies have shown both biochemical and clinical stability or even improvement in acromegaly during pregnancy.[50,51]

Diagnosis of Acromegaly During Pregnancy

The pregnancy-related changes in GH, GH variant, and IGF-1 have made the diagnosis of acromegaly challenging. In addition, the commonly used GH assays do not distinguish between pituitary GH and the placental GH variant. Moreover, both placental and pituitary GHs are not suppressed by oral glucose,[42] so oral glucose tolerance tests should not be used to diagnose acromegaly in pregnancy. Therefore, some investigators recommend waiting to diagnose acromegaly until after delivery, when the placental GH levels decrease precipitously. Pituitary MRI is usually reserved for patients with symptoms suggesting acute intracranial processes; for example, concern for pituitary apoplexy or those with known acromegaly reporting severe headache and newly developed vision defects.

Management of Acromegaly During Pregnancy

For those with mild disease and not on treatment before conception, an expectant approach can be taken because stable disease or spontaneous improvement of acromegaly has been reported during pregnancy.[45,50,51] In patients receiving medical treatment before conception, their medication should be stopped either before planned conception or immediately after confirming pregnancy.[52–55] Most patients with acromegaly who had such drug withdrawal did well during pregnancy.[43] Close monitoring of potential complications from acromegaly is warranted in these patients. In those with suspected tumor enlargement causing a visual defect or severe headache, MRI may be necessary to confirm whether an intervention is necessary.

Medical treatment during pregnancy should be reserved for patients with active acromegaly requiring treatment because of severe symptoms from large tumors; for example, severe headache, vision defects, or tumor enlargement.[52] SSAs are effective in controlling both tumor growth and IGF-1 levels in nonpregnant acromegalic patients.[55] Because SSAs cross the placenta, potentially affecting fetal brain somatostatin receptors, and decrease uterine artery blood flow, their use during pregnancy is not recommended.[56,57] Retrospective studies and small case series have shown that SSAs are generally effective and safe during pregnancy,[45,57,58] although small for gestational age[43] and shorter birth length[57] have been reported.

Dopamine agonists have been used in the treatment of pregnant women with acromegaly and are reported to be safe.[42,43,56] More safety data about the use of dopamine agonist during pregnancy are from large series involving the treatment of prolactinoma.[1,2]

Pegvisomant is a GH receptor antagonist[44,59,60] and its use during 35 pregnancies (27 maternal and 8 paternal exposure), including 3 cases in which pegvisomant was continued throughout pregnancy,[60] showed no adverse pregnancy outcomes. However, children with GH-insensitivity syndrome (Laron syndrome) caused by GH receptor abnormalities have multiple abnormalities, so pegvisomant use cannot be recommended during pregnancy.[61]

Considering the prolonged nature of the course of most patients with acromegaly, interruption of medical therapy for 9 to 12 months should not have a particularly adverse effect on the long-term outcome. In contrast, these drugs can control tumor growth and, for enlarging tumors, their reintroduction during pregnancy may be warranted versus operating. In patients with severe acromegalic symptoms not controlled by or intolerant to medical treatments, or with acute symptoms caused by tumor enlargement (eg, vision loss), or concern for pituitary apoplexy, emergent transsphenoidal surgery can be considered, preferably during the second trimester.

FUNCTIONING GONADOTROPIN-SECRETING ADENOMA IN PREGNANCY

Most gonadotroph tumors are clinically silent. Only 2 cases of functioning gonadotropin-secreting adenomas during pregnancy have been reported. In 1 case, the patient conceived naturally but developed ovarian hyperstimulation syndrome at gestation week 5 and had termination of pregnancy at the ninth week because of the development of deep vein thrombosis.[62] In the second case, the patient presented with positive pregnancy tests and markedly enlarged ovaries. Her pregnancy was terminated because of abnormal hCG levels and absent intrauterine pregnancy.[63]

THYROID-STIMULATING HORMONE–SECRETING ADENOMA IN PREGNANCY

Thyroid-stimulating hormone (TSH)–secreting pituitary adenomas are rare.[64] They are characterized by hyperthyroidism with increased free T4 and T3 levels, inappropriately normal or increased levels of TSH, and most are macroadenomas.[64] From 20% to 25% of these tumors may cosecrete GH or PRL.[65] Only 6 cases of TSH-secreting pituitary adenomas have been reported during pregnancy.[66–68] Macroadenomas were found in most cases, with occasional enlargement during pregnancy necessitating treatment.[66,67] Treatments of TSH-secreting adenomas during pregnancy were targeted to the tumor (surgery, radiation, or octreotide) and/or the hyperthyroidism with antithyroid medications.[66–69]

CLINICALLY NONFUNCTIONING PITUITARY ADENOMA IN PREGNANCY

A clinically nonfunctioning pituitary adenoma (CNFA) does not cause a clinical syndrome because of overproduction of a pituitary hormone. In the nonpregnant population, CNFAs represent about 30% to 40% of all pituitary tumors,[70,71] and most stain positive for gonadotropins.[71]

Most CNFAs remain stable in size during pregnancy,[7,38,69,70] especially those that were treated with surgery or radiotherapy before conception.[69] However, in a recent study, tumor enlargement during pregnancy was reported in 1 of 7 CNFAs diagnosed before conception and in 3 of 5 CNFAs diagnosed in pregnancy.[69] In addition, lactotroph hyperplasia during pregnancy may push the CNFAs up to affect the optic chiasm.[72] Pregnancy outcomes do not seem to be affected by CNFAs.[69] CNFAs usually do not need treatment during pregnancy. However, symptoms suggestive of tumor enlargement should be monitored, including severe headaches or vision defects. Pituitary apoplexy has been reported in CNFAs, especially macroadenomas.[69]

REFERENCES

1. Molitch ME. Prolactinoma in pregnancy. Best Pract Res Clin Endocrinol Metab 2011;25:885–96.
2. Molitch ME. Endocrinology in pregnancy: management of the pregnant patient with a prolactinoma. Eur J Endocrinol 2015;172:R205–13.
3. Casanueva FF, Molitch ME, Schlechte JA, et al. Guidelines of the Pituitary Society for the diagnosis and management of prolactinomas. Clin Endocrinol (Oxf) 2006; 65:265–73.
4. Gillam MP, Molitch ME, Lombardi G, et al. Advances in the treatment of prolactinomas. Endocr Rev 2006;27:485–534.

5. Melmed S, Casanueva FF, Hoffman AR, et al. Diagnosis and treatment of hyper-prolactinemia: an Endocrine Society clinical practice guideline. J Clin Endocrinol Metab 2011;96:273–88.

6. Stalldecker G, Mallea-Gil MS, Guitelman M, et al. Effects of cabergoline on pregnancy and embryo-fetal development: retrospective study on 103 pregnancies and a review of the literature. Pituitary 2010;13:345–50.

7. Karaca Z, Yarman S, Ozbas I, et al. How does pregnancy affect the patients with pituitary adenomas: a study on 113 pregnancies from Turkey. J Endocrinol Invest 2018;41:129–41.

8. Ono M, Miki N, Amano K, et al. Individualized high-dose cabergoline therapy for hyperprolactinemic infertility in women with micro- and macroprolactinomas. J Clin Endocrinol Metab 2010;95:2672–9.

9. Lebbe M, Hubinont C, Bernard P, et al. Outcome of 100 pregnancies initiated under treatment with cabergoline in hyperprolactinaemic women. Clin Endocrinol (Oxf) 2010;73:236–42.

10. Glezer A, Bronstein MD. Prolactinomas, cabergoline, and pregnancy. Endocrine 2014;47:64–9.

11. Webster J. A comparative review of the tolerability profiles of dopamine agonists in the treatment of hyperprolactinaemia and inhibition of lactation. Drug Saf 1996; 14:228–38.

12. Hurault-Delarue C, Montastruc JL, Beau AB, et al. Pregnancy outcome in women exposed to dopamine agonists during pregnancy: a pharmacoepidemiology study in EFEMERIS database. Arch Gynecol Obstet 2014;290:263–70.

13. Rigg LA, Lein A, Yen SS. Pattern of increase in circulating prolactin levels during human gestation. Am J Obstet Gynecol 1977;129:454–6.

14. Dinc H, Esen F, Demirci A, et al. Pituitary dimensions and volume measurements in pregnancy and post partum. MR assessment. Acta Radiol 1998;39:64–9.

15. Rastogi A, Bhadada SK, Bhansali A. Pregnancy and tumor outcomes in infertile women with macroprolactinoma on cabergoline therapy. Gynecol Endocrinol 2017;33:270–3.

16. Grand'Maison S, Weber F, Bedard MJ, et al. Pituitary apoplexy in pregnancy: a case series and literature review. Obstet Med 2015;8:177–83.

17. Domingue ME, Devuyst F, Alexopoulou O, et al. Outcome of prolactinoma after pregnancy and lactation: a study on 73 patients. Clin Endocrinol (Oxf) 2014;80: 642–8.

18. Samaan NA, Schultz PN, Leavens TA, et al. Pregnancy after treatment in patients with prolactinoma: operation versus bromocriptine. Am J Obstet Gynecol 1986; 155:1300–5.

19. Salvatori R. Surgical treatment of microprolactinomas: pros. Endocrine 2014;47: 725–9.

20. Molitch ME. Pregnancy and the hyperprolactinemic woman. N Engl J Med 1985; 312:1364–70.

21. Molitch ME. Diagnosis and treatment of pituitary adenomas: a review. JAMA 2017;317:516–24.

22. Divers WA Jr, Yen SS. Prolactin-producing microadenomas in pregnancy. Obstet Gynecol 1983;62:425–9.

23. Webb JA, Thomsen HS, Morcos SK, Members of Contrast Media Safety Committee of European Society of Urogenital Radiology (ESUR). The use of iodinated and gadolinium contrast media during pregnancy and lactation. Eur Radiol 2005;15:1234–40.

24. Ray JG, Vermeulen MJ, Bharatha A, et al. Association between MRI exposure during pregnancy and fetal and childhood outcomes. JAMA 2016;316:952–61.

25. Belchetz PE, Carty A, Clearkin LG, et al. Failure of prophylactic surgery to avert massive pituitary expansion in pregnancy. Clin Endocrinol (Oxf) 1986;25:325–30.

26. Brodsky JB, Cohen EN, Brown BW Jr, et al. Surgery during pregnancy and fetal outcome. Am J Obstet Gynecol 1980;138:1165–7.

27. Cohen-Kerem R, Railton C, Oren D, et al. Pregnancy outcome following non-obstetric surgical intervention. Am J Surg 2005;190:467–73.

28. Lindsay JR, Nieman LK. The hypothalamic-pituitary-adrenal axis in pregnancy: challenges in disease detection and treatment. Endocr Rev 2005;26:775–99.

29. Polli N, Pecori Giraldi F, Cavagnini F. Cushing's disease and pregnancy. Pituitary 2004;7:237–41.

30. Yawar A, Zuberi LM, Haque N. Cushing's disease and pregnancy: case report and literature review. Endocr Pract 2007;13:296–9.

31. Brue T, Amodru V, Castinetti F. MANAGEMENT OF ENDOCRINE DISEASE: management of Cushing's syndrome during pregnancy: solved and unsolved questions. Eur J Endocrinol 2018;178(6):R259–66.

32. Lopes LM, Francisco RP, Galletta MA, et al. Determination of nighttime salivary cortisol during pregnancy: comparison with values in non-pregnancy and Cushing's disease. Pituitary 2016;19:30–8.

33. Caimari F, Valassi E, Garbayo P, et al. Cushing's syndrome and pregnancy outcomes: a systematic review of published cases. Endocrine 2017;55:555–63.

34. Gopal RA, Acharya SV, Bandgar TR, et al. Cushing disease with pregnancy. Gynecol Endocrinol 2012;28:533–5.

35. Berwaerts J, Verhelst J, Mahler C, et al. Cushing's syndrome in pregnancy treated by ketoconazole: case report and review of the literature. Gynecol Endocrinol 1999;13:175–82.

36. Woo I, Ehsanipoor RM. Cabergoline therapy for Cushing disease throughout pregnancy. Obstet Gynecol 2013;122:485–7.

37. Boronat M, Marrero D, Lopez-Plasencia Y, et al. Successful outcome of pregnancy in a patient with Cushing's disease under treatment with ketoconazole during the first trimester of gestation. Gynecol Endocrinol 2011;27:675–7.

38. Bronstein MD, Paraiba DB, Jallad RS. Management of pituitary tumors in pregnancy. Nat Rev Endocrinol 2011;7:301–10.

39. Fleseriu M. Medical treatment of Cushing disease: new targets, new hope. Endocrinol Metab Clin North Am 2015;44:51–70.

40. Biller BM, Grossman AB, Stewart PM, et al. Treatment of adrenocorticotropin-dependent Cushing's syndrome: a consensus statement. J Clin Endocrinol Metab 2008;93:2454–62.

41. Verhaeghe J. Does the physiological acromegaly of pregnancy benefit the fetus? Gynecol Obstet Invest 2008;66:217–26.

42. Cheng V, Faiman C, Kennedy L, et al. Pregnancy and acromegaly: a review. Pituitary 2012;15:59–63.

43. Caron P, Broussaud S, Bertherat J, et al. Acromegaly and pregnancy: a retrospective multicenter study of 59 pregnancies in 46 women. J Clin Endocrinol Metab 2010;95:4680–7.

44. Cheng S, Grasso L, Martinez-Orozco JA, et al. Pregnancy in acromegaly: experience from two referral centers and systematic review of the literature. Clin Endocrinol (Oxf) 2012;76:264–71.

45. Jallad RS, Shimon I, Fraenkel M, et al. Outcome of pregnancies in a large cohort of women with acromegaly. Clin Endocrinol (Oxf) 2018;88:896–907.

46. Cozzi R, Attanasio R, Barausse M. Pregnancy in acromegaly: a one-center experience. Eur J Endocrinol 2006;155:279–84.
47. Kasuki L, Neto LV, Takiya CM, et al. Growth of an aggressive tumor during pregnancy in an acromegalic patient. Endocr J 2012;59:313–9.
48. Kupersmith MJ, Rosenberg C, Kleinberg D. Visual loss in pregnant women with pituitary adenomas. Ann Intern Med 1994;121:473–7.
49. Okada Y, Morimoto I, Ejima K, et al. A case of active acromegalic woman with a marked increase in serum insulin-like growth factor-1 levels after delivery. Endocr J 1997;44:117–20.
50. Lau SL, McGrath S, Evain-Brion D, et al. Clinical and biochemical improvement in acromegaly during pregnancy. J Endocrinol Invest 2008;31:255–61.
51. Dias M, Boguszewski C, Gadelha M, et al. Acromegaly and pregnancy: a prospective study. Eur J Endocrinol 2014;170:301–10.
52. Fleseriu M. Medical treatment of acromegaly in pregnancy, highlights on new reports. Endocrine 2015;49:577–9.
53. Bornstein SR, Allolio B, Arlt W, et al. Diagnosis and treatment of primary adrenal insufficiency: an Endocrine Society clinical practice guideline. J Clin Endocrinol Metab 2016;101:364–89.
54. Abucham J, Bronstein MD, Dias ML. Management of endocrine disease: acromegaly and pregnancy: a contemporary review. Eur J Endocrinol 2017;177: R1–12.
55. Katznelson L, Laws ER Jr, Melmed S, et al. Acromegaly: an endocrine society clinical practice guideline. J Clin Endocrinol Metab 2014;99:3933–51.
56. Muhammad A, Neggers SJ, van der Lely AJ. Pregnancy and acromegaly. Pituitary 2017;20:179–84.
57. Maffei P, Tamagno G, Nardelli GB, et al. Effects of octreotide exposure during pregnancy in acromegaly. Clin Endocrinol (Oxf) 2010;72:668–77.
58. Mikhail N. Octreotide treatment of acromegaly during pregnancy. Mayo Clin Proc 2002;77:297–8.
59. Brian SR, Bidlingmaier M, Wajnrajch MP, et al. Treatment of acromegaly with pegvisomant during pregnancy: maternal and fetal effects. J Clin Endocrinol Metab 2007;92:3374–7.
60. van der Lely AJ, Gomez R, Heissler JF, et al. Pregnancy in acromegaly patients treated with pegvisomant. Endocrine 2015;49:769–73.
61. Laron Z. Lessons from 50 years of study of Laron syndrome. Endocr Pract 2015; 21:1395–402.
62. Baba T, Endo T, Kitajima Y, et al. Spontaneous ovarian hyperstimulation syndrome and pituitary adenoma: incidental pregnancy triggers a catastrophic event. Fertil Steril 2009;92:390.e1-3.
63. Ghayuri M, Liu JH. Ovarian hyperstimulation syndrome caused by pituitary gonadotroph adenoma secreting follicle-stimulating hormone. Obstet Gynecol 2007; 109:547–9.
64. Amlashi FG, Tritos NA. Thyrotropin-secreting pituitary adenomas: epidemiology, diagnosis, and management. Endocrine 2016;52:427–40.
65. Beck-Peccoz P, Lania A, Beckers A, et al. 2013 European thyroid association guidelines for the diagnosis and treatment of thyrotropin-secreting pituitary tumors. Eur Thyroid J 2013;2:76–82.
66. Caron P, Gerbeau C, Pradayrol L, et al. Successful pregnancy in an infertile woman with a thyrotropin-secreting macroadenoma treated with somatostatin analog (octreotide). J Clin Endocrinol Metab 1996;81:1164–8.

67. Chaiamnuay S, Moster M, Katz MR, et al. Successful management of a pregnant woman with a TSH secreting pituitary adenoma with surgical and medical therapy. Pituitary 2003;6:109–13.
68. Perdomo CM, Arabe JA, Idoate MA, et al. Management of a pregnant woman with thyrotropinoma: a case report and review of the literature. Gynecol Endocrinol 2017;33:188–92.
69. Lambert K, Rees K, Seed PT, et al. Macroprolactinomas and nonfunctioning pituitary adenomas and pregnancy outcomes. Obstet Gynecol 2017;129:185–94.
70. Araujo PB, Vieira Neto L, Gadelha MR. Pituitary tumor management in pregnancy. Endocrinol Metab Clin North Am 2015;44:181–97.
71. Huang W, Molitch ME. Management of nonfunctioning pituitary adenomas (NFAs): observation. Pituitary 2018;21:162–7.
72. Molitch ME. Pituitary tumors and pregnancy. Growth Horm IGF Res 2003; 13(Suppl A):S38–44.
73. Gemzell C, Wang CF. Outcome of pregnancy in women with pituitary adenoma. Fertil Steril 1979;31:363–72.
74. Holmgren U, Bergstrand G, Hagenfeldt K, et al. Women with prolactinoma – effect of pregnancy and lactation on serum prolactin and on tumour growth. Acta Endocrinol 1986;111:452–9.
75. Ampudia X, Puig-Domingo M, Schwarzstein D, et al. Outcome and long-term effects of pregnancy in women with hyperprolactinemia. Eur J Obstet Gynecol Reprod Biol 1992;46(2-3):101–7.
76. Rossi AM, Vilska S, Heinonen PK. Outcome of pregnancies in women with treated or untreated hyperprolactinemia. Eur J Obstet Gynecol Reprod Biol 1995;63: 143–6.
77. Badawy SZ, Marziale JC, Rosenbaum AE, et al. The long-term effects of pregnancy and bromocriptine tratment on prolactinomas – the value of radiologic studies. Early Pregnancy 1997;3(4):306–11.
78. Mallmann ES, Nagcl A, Spritzer PM. Pregnancy in hyperprolactinemic women. Acta Obstet Gynecol Scand 2002;81:265–7.
79. Bronstein MD, Salgado LR, Musolino NR. Medical management of pituitary adenomas: the special case of management of the pregnant woman. Pituitary 2002; 5:99–107.
80. Auriemma RS, Perone Y, Di Sarno A, et al. Results of a single-center 10-year observational survey study on recurrence of hyperprolactinemia after pregnancy and lactation. J Clin Endocrinol Metab 2013;98(1):372–9.

Other Pituitary Conditions and Pregnancy

Philippe Chanson, MD[a,b,*]

KEYWORDS

- Hypophysitis • Sheehan syndrome • Pregnancy • Diabetes insipidus
- Hypopituitarism • Autoimmune

KEY POINTS

- Lymphocytic hypophysitis (LH) may occur in the peripartum period. At present, its diagnosis is based on clinical and neuroradiological data and does not require a biopsy.
- The course of LH, in terms of mass effect, is generally spontaneously favorable but may require the administration of corticosteroids or even transsphenoidal resection.
- The course of pituitary deficiencies is highly variable; some cases recover over time, whereas others persist indefinitely.
- Sheehan syndrome is very rare in developed countries. Because agalactia and amenorrhea often are neglected, the diagnosis is generally delayed for many years.
- Diabetes insipidus occurring in late pregnancy is caused by the increased placental production of vasopressinase and disappears after delivery.

INTRODUCTION

Pituitary adenoma is the main pituitary disease that causes problems during pregnancy. However, other pituitary conditions may be detected during or complicate pregnancy. The most frequent condition is lymphocytic hypophysitis (LH), which occurs de novo during pregnancy or in the postpartum period; in developed countries it is now much more common than the classic Sheehan syndrome, which is rarely encountered because of progress in obstetrics. In addition, other tumors of the region, such as craniopharyngiomas or meningiomas, very rarely cause problems during pregnancy. Diabetes insipidus (DI) is another issue that may complicate pregnancy.

Disclosure: The author has nothing to disclose in relation to this article.
[a] Assistance Publique-Hôpitaux de Paris (P.C.), Hôpitaux Universitaires Paris-Sud, Hôpital de Bicêtre, Service d'Endocrinologie et des Maladies de la Reproduction, Centre de Référence des Maladies Rares de l'Hypophyse, 78 rue du Général Leclerc, Le Kremlin-Bicêtre F-94275, France;
[b] UMR S-1185, Fac Med Paris-Sud, Université Paris-Saclay, Le Kremlin-Bicêtre F-94276, France
* Service d'Endocrinologie et des Maladies de la Reproduction, Hôpital de Bicêtre, 78 rue du Général Leclerc, Le Kremlin-Bicêtre F-94275, France.
E-mail address: philippe.chanson@bct.aphp.fr

Endocrinol Metab Clin N Am 48 (2019) 583–603
https://doi.org/10.1016/j.ecl.2019.05.005
0889-8529/19/© 2019 Elsevier Inc. All rights reserved.

endo.theclinics.com

LYMPHOCYTIC HYPOPHYSITIS

LH is a primary autoimmune endocrinopathy that is mainly encountered in women and often detected during the last month of pregnancy or the first 2 months of the postpartum period.[1] It is a rare condition ($\approx$0.8% of pituitary lesions that are surgically removed).[2] Hypophysitis has been the subject of many recent excellent reviews.[1–6] LH is the most common histologic type of primary hypophysitis and is characterized by a diffuse infiltration of the pituitary gland with T and B lymphocytes.[1,7] According to the extent of infiltration, lymphocytic adenohypophysitis (LAH) may be observed if it involves only the anterior pituitary, lymphocytic infundibuloneurohypophysitis (LINH) if it involves the pituitary stalk and posterior pituitary, or lymphocytic panhypophysitis (LPH) if both tissues are involved.[1,4] LH is typically associated with pregnancy and was reported to be detected in 50% of cases, according to an older publication,[1] but this high prevalence was not reported in 3 more recent case series, in which 24%, 10%, or even fewer cases of LH were associated with pregnancy in female patients.[8–11] This discrepancy may be caused by an increased awareness that this condition may occur in nonpregnant patients and that MRI features of LH are increasingly being recognized.[12]

Clinical Presentation

The first case was described by Goudie and Pinkerton[13] in the early 60s of a 22-year-old woman who died of a postpartum adrenal crisis. Since the first case of LH was authenticated by a pituitary biopsy in 1987,[14] several hundred cases that have been confirmed by a pathologic study have been published.[15] However, currently, the condition is typically diagnosed without the pathologic proof, particularly in the context of pregnancy, and new cases are no longer being published. Similar to other autoimmune diseases, LH predominates in women (80% of cases), and most cases are observed in women of reproductive age. The clinical presentation of LH in the context of pregnancy is typical. At the end of pregnancy, the woman complains of signs and symptoms suggestive of a pituitary mass effect, including headaches and alterations of visual acuity and the visual field that are induced by the compression of the optic chiasm[1,2,16,17] **(Table 1)**. More rarely, oculomotor palsy indicates an impact on the cavernous sinus.[18–22] All these signs and symptoms, which usually suggest the presence of a pituitary macroadenoma (and may evoke, in particular, a pituitary apoplexy), should prompt the clinician to require imaging of the hypothalamic-pituitary region.

In the postpartum period, hypophysitis presents more frequently with signs of pituitary deficiency. This condition may be observed in an acute setting in which a corticotropic deficiency is responsible for weight loss, severe fatigue, pallor, hyponatremia, or even symptoms and signs of adrenal crisis leading to cardiovascular shock (vasoplegic shock).[23] The more progressive clinical forms combine corticotropic (fatigue, pallor, and weight loss) and gonadotropic (amenorrhea) deficiencies. This combined deficiency is responsible for a severe androgen deficiency marked by the progressive disappearance of axillary and pubic hair, which is suggestive of an anterior pituitary insufficiency. When cortisol deficiency is associated with growth hormone (GH) deficiency, hypoglycemia may be observed, particularly during fasting. The gonadotropic deficiency, which is masked during pregnancy, may manifest only in the postpartum period as amenorrhea. This type of hypogonadotropic hypogonadism is most often transient,[24] but partial or severe chronic gonadotropic deficiencies have been described. In rare cases, gonadotropic deficiency may also be secondary to hyperprolactinemia related to a stalk effect (hypothalamic-pituitary disconnection) mediated by the infiltration or compression of the pituitary stalk. In contrast, a prolactin (PRL)

Table 1
Differential diagnosis of lymphocytic hypophysitis, Sheehan syndrome, and nonfunctioning pituitary adenoma in the acute phase at time of pregnancy or postpartum

	LH	Pituitary Nonfunctioning Pituitary Adenoma	Sheehan Syndrome
Frequency among pituitary lesions occurring during pregnancy	Most frequent	Very rare	Extremely rare
Presentation			
Headache	+++	+	No
Visual problems	+	+	No
Agalactia	Sometimes	No	Always
Galactorrhea	Sometimes	Sometimes	Never
Signs of adrenal crisis (hyponatremia, shock)	Sometimes	Never	Always
DI	20%	Never	Never
Previous History			
Autoimmune diseases	Yes	No	No
Infertility	No	Yes	No
Context of massive obstetric hemorrhage	No	No	Yes
Pituitary Function			
Gonadotropic deficiency	+	++	+++
Thyrotropic deficiency	++	+	++
Corticotropic deficiency	+++	+	++
Panhypopituitarism	++	+	Yes
Hyperprolactinemia	+	++	Never
PRL deficiency	Sometimes	Never	Always
Posterior pituitary function	DI (20%)	Never	Minor disturbances
Neuroradiology			
Unilateral depression of sella floor	No	Yes	No
Enlarged pituitary fossa	No	Yes	No
Contrast enhancement	+++	++	++
Lateralized lesion	No	Yes	No
Diffuse enlargement of the gland	+++	No (pituitary gland visible besides the lesion)	++
Posterior pituitary bright spot	Not visible in case of DI	Always visible	Always visible
Pituitary stalk thickening	++	No	No
Dural enhancement	+	No	No
Signs of hemorrhage/necrosis	Sometimes	Rare (unless pituitary apoplexy)	Always

Abbreviation: PRL, prolactin.

Data from Honegger J, Giese S. Acute pituitary disease in pregnancy: how to handle hypophysitis and Sheehan's syndrome. *Minerva Endocrinol.* 2018;43(4):465-475 and Karaca Z, Kelestimur F. Pregnancy and other pituitary disorders (including GH deficiency). *Best Pract Res Clin Endocrinol Metab.* 2011;25(6):897-910.

deficiency is occasionally responsible for the failure to lactate, which, when associated with amenorrhea, strongly confirms the diagnosis.[25]

Posterior pituitary involvement (in LINH or LPH), which is manifested as DI, is rare in patients with pregnancy-related LH.[26,27] It is sometimes masked by an associated corticotropic deficit, in which case the occurrence of polyuria and polydipsia at the time of glucocorticoid substitution allows the clinician to diagnose a vasopressin deficiency. The presence of DI helps the clinician differentiate LH from nonfunctioning pituitary adenomas (NFPAs) because, except in the very rare cases of pituitary apoplexy, pituitary adenomas are almost never associated with DI.

Biochemical Evaluation

A suspicion of LH requires an evaluation of all pituitary axes and the identification of signs of DI. More than 70% of patients with primary LH are diagnosed with complete or partial hypopituitarism, whereas 20% have DI[1] (see **Table 1**). Corticotropic axis involvement is the most common type; it affects 60% of patients with LH[2,15] and explains the potential severity of the disease by the risk of adrenal crisis and eventually death.[13,24,28,29] It is most often severe, because plasma concentrations of adrenocorticotropic hormone (ACTH) and cortisol are very low and unresponsive to stimulation tests. Notably, ACTH deficiency can be isolated.[1,3] Hyperprolactinemia, usually less than 100 ng/mL, is observed in 30% to 40% of patients with LH (whether or not it is associated with pregnancy).[3,8,10,30,31] Hyperprolactinemia is difficult to differentiate from physiologic hyperprolactinemia of pregnancy and postpartum hyperprolactinemia, and from hyperprolactinemia related to a stalk interruption by an NFPA,[32] which explains the poor diagnostic value of this biochemical parameter in this context.[25] In contrast, the PRL deficiency, which is much more suggestive of hypophysitis, is usually severe, and PRL levels in these patients are often very low.[1,25]

Gonadotropic axis involvement, which is responsible for postpartum amenorrhea, affects half of all women. Thyrotropic hormone deficiency has been described in half of patients with LH.[15] When it occurs, it is often severe and is characterized by very low FT4 levels that are associated with very low or even undetectable thyroid-stimulating hormone (TSH) concentrations (which is not encountered in patients with NFPAs, in which TSH concentrations are generally in the normal range), indicating the direct destruction of pituitary thyrotrophs.[33] However, low FT4 levels with normal or moderately increased (usually <6–10 mIU/L) TSH levels may be observed. GH deficiency is often less well documented in these patients but seems to be common.[2,34] Panhypopituitarism is frequently observed at the time of diagnosis.[2,3,16]

The true prevalence of each pituitary deficiency is difficult to assess in patients with pregnancy-related LH, because it depends on the time when the evaluation is performed. Pituitary deficiencies may completely or partially recover over time.[17,34,35]

Neuroradiological Aspects

MRI of coronal and sagittal sections of the pituitary region using T1-weighted (T1W) and T2-weighted (T2W) sequences is crucial for the diagnosis. A gadolinium injection is not recommended during pregnancy, but it may be proposed in the postpartum period. During the active phase of the disease, the most frequently observed neuroradiological aspect is a pseudotumor lesion (**Fig. 1**),[5,9,12,25,34,36–38] and the appearance may resemble a pituitary adenoma. However, the sella floor is horizontal and the borders of the sella turcica are normal (discussed later). Before gadolinium injection, T1 images usually show a homogeneous symmetric mass of the pituitary region that typically presents an isointense or sometimes hypointense or hyperintense signal, often

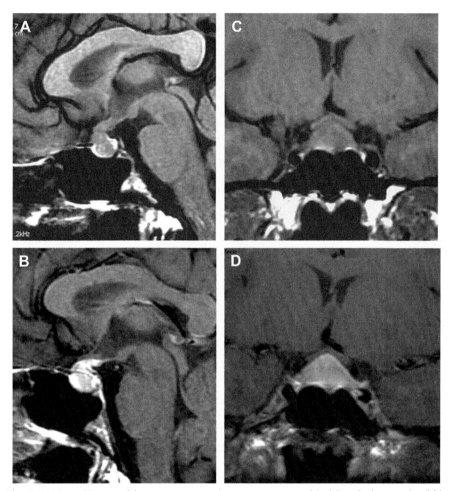

Fig. 1. LH in a 27-year-old woman presenting severe retro-orbital headache on the fifth month of pregnancy. Sagittal (*A, B*) and coronal (*C, D*) T1W sections before (*A, C*) and after (*B, D*) gadolinium injection showing a triangular symmetric pituitary mass with superior extension along the pituitary stalk, strongly enhanced after injection, compressing the optic chiasm. (*From* Bonneville JF, Bonneville F, Cattin F, et al. MRI of the Pituitary Gland. Springer International: Publishing Switzerland 2016.)

with a suprasellar expansion that may compress the optic chiasm (see **Fig. 1**). The triangular aspect of the suprasellar expansion, although inconsistent, is very suggestive of hypophysitis. The mass is homogeneously hyperintense on T2W sections (**Fig. 2**). When the lesion infiltrates the pituitary stalk, an enlargement of the latter or obliteration of the lower recess of the third ventricle are observed, all strongly evoking a diagnosis of LINH (**Fig. 3**). However, these LINH forms are less frequent during pregnancy or in the postpartum period than in patients with non–pregnancy-related LH.[24] The presence of DI is associated with the disappearance of the posterior pituitary bright spot.[39–41]

After the injection of gadolinium, a very intense, often homogeneous enhancement of contrast is observed. This hypersignal, which is more important than the signal that is typically observed in pituitary adenomas, is a characteristic finding.

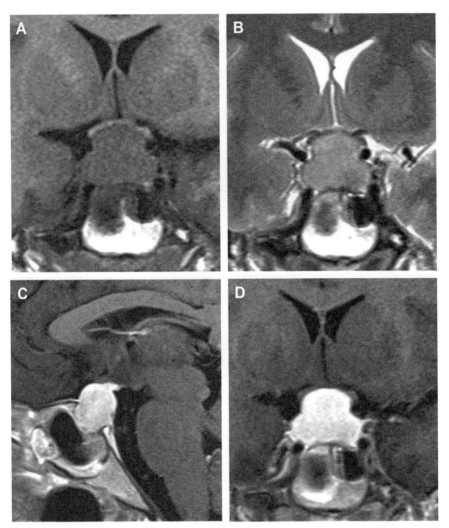

Fig. 2. Postpartum LH revealed by severe headaches, fatigue, and hypotension. Coronal T1W (*A*), and T2W (*B*) sections and sagittal (*C*) and coronal (*D*) T1W sections after gadolinium injection showing a large pituitary mass, hypointense on T1W and hyperintense on T2W sections, symmetric with suprasellar extension, strongly enhanced after injection, and compressing the optic chiasm. (*From* Bonneville JF, Bonneville F, Cattin F, et al. MRI of the Pituitary Gland. Springer International: Publishing Switzerland 2016.)

Sometimes, this hyperintense signal surrounds the mass, giving it a crown appearance that can infiltrate the dura[12,42] and the cavernous sinus.[18–22] The lymphoplasmacytic infiltration of the latter explains the oculomotor impairments. Since the advent of MRI, computed tomography (CT) scan of the pituitary region, which is less efficient at visualizing infiltrative lesions, has been used less frequently. Its only indication in this context is to improve the visualization of the bony limits of the sella turcica in patients with a tumor mass. CT shows the absence of erosion of the walls and persistence of the horizontal floor of the sella, which are more suggestive of LH than a pituitary adenoma.

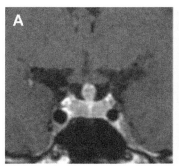
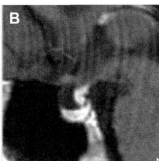

Fig. 3. Infundibuloneurohypophysitis. Coronal (*A*) and sagittal (*B*) T1W sections after gadolinium injection showing the strong enhancement of the lesion limited to infundibulum, pituitary stalk, and neurohypophysis. (*Courtesy of* JF Bonneville, Liege, Belgium.)

Course of the Disease

Given the lack of homogeneity of descriptions and follow-up of cases reported in the literature, a schematic of the natural history of LH is difficult to construct. According to the published cases, in the absence of any treatment, the pseudotumor process generally regresses spontaneously and the pituitary gland subsequently atrophies, which results in an empty sella on MRI[35,43–46] (**Fig. 4**). Researchers have not clearly determined whether the course is improved by corticosteroid treatment. In terms of pituitary functions, the course is very variable, with complete or partial recovery of initial panhypopituitarism, worsening of anterior pituitary insufficiency, and the onset of a new deficit or DI.[17,24,30,35,43–45,47,48]

In general, peripartum LH does not recur in a subsequent pregnancy.[35,44,45,49] Very few recurrences during successive pregnancies have been reported.[24,49] Thus, when LH has occurred in a first pregnancy, a contraindication for another pregnancy does not exist and, if gonadotropic failure persists after LH, ovulation induction may be proposed.

Pathology

The pathology varies according to the stage of the disease.[1,3,4] From a macroscopic perspective, in the acute period, the pituitary gland appears to be enlarged and its

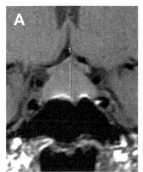
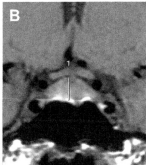
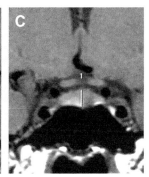

Fig. 4. Spontaneous course of a LH in the same patient as **Fig. 1**. T1W sections at diagnosis (*A*), 2 months (*B*), and 6 months later (*C*), showing the progressive normalization of the sellar content, with the decrease in the height (1) of the lesion. (*From* Bonneville JF, Bonneville F, Cattin F, et al. MRI of the Pituitary Gland. Springer International: Publishing Switzerland 2016.)

consistency is generally soft but is sometimes more fibrous; infiltration often involves the dura mater, which is very adherent, as are the surrounding structures. Afterward, the pituitary becomes atrophic and presents fibrosis. According to the pathology, the surgically resected or biopsied pituitary mass is extensively infiltrated by lymphocytes that may organize in lymphoid follicles[1,3]; plasma cells may also be detected and are more rarely accompanied by eosinophils, macrophages, and neutrophils (**Fig. 5**). Lymphocyte infiltration may be associated with foci of necrosis and sometimes granulomas or isolated multinucleated giant cells.

Association with Other Autoimmune Diseases and Circulating Pituitary Antibodies

LH clearly has an autoimmune origin. Its association with other autoimmune diseases is reported in 25% to 50% of cases.[17,24,30,35,43–45,47,48] These conditions can precede or, on the contrary, occur long after LH. Autoimmune thyroid diseases, such as Hashimoto or silent thyroiditis, or even Graves disease, are the most frequent; Addison disease, type 1 diabetes mellitus, hypoparathyroidism, and nonendocrine autoimmune diseases such as atrophic gastritis, systemic erythematosus lupus, or Sjögren syndrome have also been reported. LH occasionally occurs in the context of autoimmune polyendocrine syndrome type I/autoimmune polyendocrinopathy-candidiasis-ectodermal dystrophy.[50]

Given the autoimmune nature of this condition, several groups have sought to identify circulating antibodies against the pituitary gland to provide clinicians with a noninvasive diagnostic method without resorting to a surgical pituitary biopsy. These antibodies have primarily been investigated using indirect immunofluorescence and immunoblotting of human, primate, rodent, or established cell lines as the target tissue.[4,46,51–54] However, to date, the sensitivity and specificity of antipituitary antibody detection methods are insufficient for use in routine clinical practice.[36,55–57] Future research focused on identifying the pituitary antigens is needed to improve the performance of these diagnostic tests.

Differential Diagnosis

Ultimately the diagnosis of LH may require histologic proof in a sample obtained by surgery or biopsy, but the presumptive diagnosis of LH is generally based on clinical, hormonal, and neuroradiological findings and allows the patient to avoid the risks of surgery, particularly in the context of pregnancy.[16,36] During pregnancy, LH may mimic a nonfunctioning pituitary macroadenoma. The respective features of each

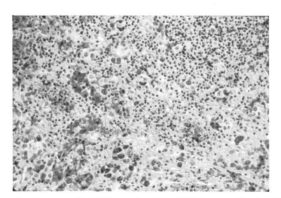

Fig. 5. Diffuse lymphoplasmacytic infiltrate typical of LH in a patient with pituitary mass, which was biopsied (hematoxylin-eosin, original magnification ×64).

condition help clinicians make a presumptive diagnosis, as has been reported in detail from both a clinical[25] and neuroradiological[12,37] perspective. These features are summarized in **Table 1**. In general, patients who present with pituitary adenomas have a history of infertility, whereas normal fertility occurs in patients with LH. Visual disturbances and headaches seem to be more frequent in patients with LH. Lower PRL levels are detected in patients with LH compared with patients with pituitary adenomas. Abnormalities in thyroid and/or adrenal function are also more common in patients with LH.[25] Imaging helps clinicians distinguish between these conditions (discussed earlier), as summarized in **Table 1**.

Most likely, the most important argument in favor of LH is the occurrence of a mass effect during pregnancy. NFPAs are rarely observed in young women and are not prone to increase in size during pregnancy. Macroprolactinomas may increase in size during pregnancy and may also be a differential diagnosis, but the levels of PRL associated with macroprolactinomas are clearly higher than in normal pregnancy or patients with hyperprolactinemia related to stalk effect of LH. Moreover, macroprolactinomas are generally responsible for infertility and thus they are generally diagnosed before pregnancy rather than during pregnancy.[58]

In the postpartum period, failure to lactate is generally a sign of LH rather than a pituitary adenoma.[25] At that time, as during pregnancy, the differential diagnosis of LH may also be a nonfunctioning pituitary macroadenoma or pituitary apoplexy, or, alternatively, Sheehan syndrome.[16,38,59–62] Sheehan syndrome results from a pituitary infarction related to massive peripartum hemorrhage and/or shock at the time of delivery (discussed later). In the absence of this massive hemorrhagic context, the diagnosis of Sheehan syndrome is easily excluded. When the diagnosis of pituitary insufficiency is made during the chronic phase, long after delivery and retrospectively, because the onset of symptoms dates back to the postpartum period, the differential diagnosis between LH and Sheehan syndrome may be more confusing. The absence of hemorrhagic shock at the time of delivery favors the diagnosis of LH rather than Sheehan syndrome (**Table 1**).

DI is a condition leading to the detection of several tumors and infiltration of the hypothalamus-pituitary region. These tumors include cranopharyngiomas, meningiomas (which may increase in size during pregnancy; discussed later), and pituitary metastases, neurosarcoidosis, histiocytosis, and tuberculosis. In cases presenting a mass effect, these diseases, therefore, are always discussed because they may occur during pregnancy and in the postpartum period, and may result in hypopituitarism associated with posterior pituitary involvement.[63–65] In contrast, pituitary adenomas are almost never responsible for DI.

In addition, very few cases of primary granulomatous hypophysitis related to pregnancy and proved by a pituitary biopsy have also been reported.[66,67]

Management

The management of patients with LH, which includes watchful waiting, corticosteroids, or surgery, varies according to the clinical presentation and spontaneous course.

Nevertheless, clinicians must consider that each patient with LH may have a corticotropic deficiency (with the risk of adrenal crisis) or may present with DI (with the risk of dehydration). Both may be assessed (discussed earlier) and treated adequately. Obviously, an evaluation and treatment of thyrotropic deficiency are also mandatory.[68]

In general, as soon as the diagnosis of LH is made (from an in-depth MRI analysis and hormonal evaluation designed to exclude an NFPA; discussed earlier), the patient is managed conservatively. The spontaneous course is usually favorable, not only in terms of the mass effect but also in terms of the pituitary insufficiency, which may recover in one-third of cases.[16] If the diagnosis is made during pregnancy, clinicians argue for avoiding any treatment and choosing watchful waiting. When headaches are tolerable or vision problems are minor, patients may also be managed conservatively as long as their regular and close monitoring reveals stabilization or improvement, particularly if the expected date of delivery is close and allows the patient to wait for a short period of time. A spontaneous improvement of vision problems has been observed in some patients who are treated conservatively.[69,70] In cases of severe or worsening vision problems or intolerable headaches, a trial period of glucocorticoid treatment can be established if the diagnosis of LH is certain. This treatment facilitates a rapid improvement in most cases, but recurrence of symptoms seems to be frequent after treatment withdrawal.[18,71–73]

Surgery via the transsphenoidal route has long been considered the treatment of choice, particularly in the postpartum period. It improves vision problems and headaches in almost all patients. Nevertheless, the improvement in the ability to diagnose LH without the need for a biopsy has reduced the need for surgery, particularly in the context of pregnancy or the postpartum period.[36] When LH occurs at the end of pregnancy and is complicated by severe symptoms, clinicians may recommend that delivery is accelerated by inducing labor or performing a cesarean section rather than operating on the pituitary.[16,49,74,75] Surgery is now reserved for the difficult cases in which the differential diagnosis from an NFPA or other tumor is impossible; when observation only or the use of glucocorticoids does not allow the patient to wait for a spontaneous improvement; or if mass symptoms, particularly vision problems or headaches, worsen. A preferred option seems to be to postpone surgery after delivery if symptoms are moderate and stable. This type of surgery requires a skilled surgeon to limit the excision and allow vision defects to improve while avoiding radical resection of the lesion, which would lead to postoperative panhypopituitarism and often DI. The babies are generally healthy at birth and do not present specific problems.

SHEEHAN SYNDROME

Sheehan syndrome is extremely rare in developed countries (0.2–2.8 cases per 100,000 women),[76] whereas it is frequent in less developed countries,[62] reaching a prevalence of 3.1% in Kashmir,[77] where it may be associated with maternal death and is one of the major causes of hypopituitarism.

Sheehan syndrome occurs secondary to an infarction of the normal pituitary caused by massive peripartum hemorrhage and/or shock during or soon after childbirth.

Clinical Presentation and Diagnosis

The observation of a massive postpartum hemorrhage or shock is required to differentiate Sheehan syndrome from peripartum hypophysitis (see **Table 1**).[76,78]

However, the diagnosis of Sheehan syndrome is generally delayed by a dozen years[62,76–78] because hypopituitarism, which is often partial, may be only responsible for nonspecific signs and symptoms (fatigue, anemia, and so forth). These symptoms are considered related to the baby blues syndrome or postpartum depression because amenorrhea is masked by the early resumption of oral contraception and/or because the diagnostic value of agalactia is not considered an important sign. Moreover, even after severe hemorrhaging, the occurrence of Sheehan syndrome is rare.[79] In addition, pituitary deficiency may continue to progress over many years in some patients, explaining the diagnostic delay.[62,77]

In almost all cases, the patient presents postpartum agalactia that prevents her from breastfeeding her baby, followed by amenorrhea. The usual signs and symptoms of hypopituitarism develop progressively.[68,80] The diagnosis is often made very late in a female patient who has been diagnosed with hypopituitarism and whose history reveals that she was considered as having so-called early menopause since her last pregnancy, which was terminated in the context of massive hemorrhage.

Hormonal Evaluation

The gonadotropic axis is impaired in all patients with this condition.[62] Similarly, the somatotropic axis is impaired and alterations in the thyrotropic, corticotropic, and lactotropic axes are observed in 90%, 72%, and 72% of patients, respectively.[62] In contrast, DI is rare and, if it exists, is partial.[81] In patients diagnosed with agalactia, measurements of PRL levels are useful, even years after delivery.[16] A serum PRL level less than 4.0 ng/mL is associated with lactation failure, whereas a level greater than 7.8 ng/mL is associated with normal breastfeeding.[76] In patients with a PRL deficiency, a complete evaluation of anterior pituitary hormone levels might be useful.[16]

Imaging

If imaging is performed early after the occurrence of the pituitary infarction, the pituitary gland appears enlarged (**Fig. 6**). Thereafter, progressive atrophy of the pituitary gland is observed[62] and, generally, an empty sella is detected at the time of diagnosis (**Fig. 7**).

Management

If the diagnosis is made during the acute phase, a high dose of glucocorticoids is required in parallel with hemodynamic management, blood replacement, and hemostatic surgical procedures.

SELLAR OR PARASELLAR TUMORS OTHER THAN PITUITARY ADENOMAS AND PREGNANCY

Because craniopharyngiomas are often associated with panhypopituitarism and infertility, spontaneous pregnancy is rare in patients with these tumors. Ovulation

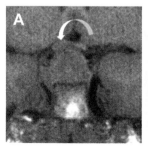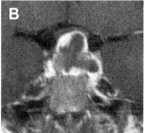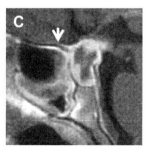

Fig. 6. Acute Sheehan syndrome in a 38-year-old woman with massive uterine hemorrhage and shock on the second day postpartum. Coronal T1W section (*A*) showing an enlarged hypointense mass abutting the optic chiasm (*curved arrow*) with a peripheral rim of enhancement after injection on T1W coronal (*B*) and sagittal (*C*) sections. Note the dural enhancement (*short arrow*) and thickening of sphenoid sinus mucosa. (*From* Bonneville JF, Bonneville F, Cattin F, et al. MRI of the Pituitary Gland. Springer International: Publishing Switzerland 2016.)

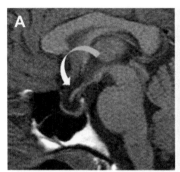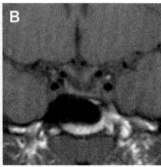

Fig. 7. Retrospective diagnosis of Sheehan syndrome in a 57-year-old woman with panhypopituitarism and previous history of massive hemorrhage at time of delivery, 20 years before. Sagittal (*A*) and coronal (*B*) T1W sections showing an aspect of empty sella. The curved arrow indicates the optic chiasm. (*From* Bonneville JF, Bonneville F, Cattin F, et al. MRI of the Pituitary Gland. Springer International: Publishing Switzerland 2016.)

may need to be induced with gonadotropins to achieve pregnancy in these patients,[82] and this procedure is generally reserved for patients without a tumor burden. If a patient is diagnosed with a craniopharyngioma before pregnancy, the tumor may increase in size (sometimes, it even may be revealed during pregnancy): this condition is very rare because, to our knowledge, less than 10 cases have been reported to date.[83–91]

Meningiomas are among the most common benign skull base tumors occurring during pregnancy.[92–96] These tumors grow during pregnancy because they often express progesterone receptors[97,98] and become sensitive to the substantial increase in sex steroid levels observed during that period. When located in the suprasellar or parasellar region, they may be responsible for vision problems and/or visual palsy.[95,99]

Because of the risk of surgery to the fetus,[100] pregnant women are typically treated conservatively, and, when possible, surgical resection of the tumor is postponed until after delivery. Preterm delivery before surgery may be appropriate early in the third term if the patient's neurologic status continues to deteriorate.[95] If the presentation is emergent and surgery is required, it is preferably performed via the transsphenoidal route.[99] The ideal trimester for surgery is the second trimester.[92]

DIABETES INSIPIDUS IN PREGNANCY

The onset of DI during pregnancy is very rare (approximately 4 cases per 100,000 pregnancies),[101] but the true prevalence is probably higher because many cases are likely undiagnosed, because of partial DI or because the diagnosis is overlooked by obstetricians.

By definition, patients with DI eliminate large quantities (>2–2.5 L/24 h) of hypotonic, hypo-osmolar urine (<250–300 mOsm/kg H_2O).[102–106]

Water Homeostasis During Pregnancy

From the seventh week of gestation, the placenta produces vasopressinase, an aminopeptidase, which inactivates endogenous arginine vasopressin (AVP).[107–109] Its maximum concentration is reached during the third trimester.[109–112] AVP degradation plateaus at 22 to 24 weeks of pregnancy through delivery, resulting in a compensatory increase in AVP synthesis and secretion.[111,113]

Serum vasopressinase activity correlates with placental weight and is higher in women with multiple pregnancies.[114]

Vasopressinase concentrations decrease substantially after delivery.

Diagnosis of Diabetes Insipidus in Pregnant Women with Hypotonic Polyuria

An investigation of a polyurodipsic state during pregnancy must first establish that it occurs secondary to hypotonic polyuria and not to osmotic polyuria (glycosuria or hypercalciuria).[115] Urine osmolarity is low (<300 mOsm/L), in contrast with high plasma osmolality (>280 mOsm/L) and high serum sodium levels (often >140 mmol/L) are observed, which, in the context of pregnancy, is unusual (natremia is usually in the lower range of normal during pregnancy).

If hypotonic polyuria is confirmed, then primary polydipsia can be rapidly excluded in the absence of psychiatric disorders, and a diagnosis of authentic DI is thus achievable. Measurement of AVP is not contributive, and the value of a copeptin assay has not been reported in this context of pregnancy.[106,116] A water deprivation test is not indicated during pregnancy because of the risk of dehydration, hypernatremia, neurologic disorders, and fetal harm.

Central DI is confirmed by the therapeutic efficacy of dDAVP (desmopressin, Minirin), which increases urine osmolarity and reduces diuresis. Nephrogenic DI is accompanied by high AVP or copeptin concentrations and does not respond to dDAVP.

The hypothesis of DI (regardless of its cause) should also be proposed in patients with unexplained polyhydramnios.[117,118]

Etiologic Diagnosis of Diabetes Insipidus During Pregnancy

Transient diabetes insipidus of pregnancy

Transient DI of pregnancy, or gestational DI, usually occurs during the third trimester. It is the most common form of DI occurring during pregnancy[107,119] and is therefore the first diagnosis to be considered.

Transient DI of pregnancy is associated with an increased vasopressinase concentration[120,121] secondary to an increase in placental production, such as in patients with multiple pregnancies or impaired hepatic vasopressinase degradation caused by preeclampsia, eclampsia, or the HELLP (hemolysis, elevated liver enzymes, and low platelet count) syndrome.[119,122–127]

Vasopressinase activity usually decreases after delivery and becomes undetectable within 5 to 6 weeks of the postpartum period.[128]

Cases of isolated DI occurring in the immediate postpartum period and not at the end of pregnancy have also been described, which are again related to an increase in vasopressinase activity.[128] This situation must be distinguished from DI associated with Sheehan syndrome (very rare) or with LH (discussed earlier), both of which are associated with other pituitary disorders and persist after delivery.

Symptoms of gestational DI resolve spontaneously in the weeks following delivery, further confirming the diagnosis of transient DI of pregnancy.[125] Transient DI does not usually recur during subsequent pregnancies.

Central diabetes insipidus during pregnancy

During normal pregnancy, AVP release is increased to maintain water reabsorption and subsequently prevent polyuria. However, if AVP secretion is abnormal because of subclinical DI caused either by neuroinfundibulitis of pregnancy or by a preexisting condition, the pregnancy can unmask polyuria and polydipsia.[129]

Common causes of central DI include tumors, pituitary infiltrations, sequelae of infundibulitis, and genetic abnormalities.[106] DI during pregnancy may reveal suprasellar lesions, such as craniopharyngiomas.[85,86]

Differential Diagnosis

Caused by AVP resistance, nephrogenic DI may be familial (associated with mutations of the AVP or aquaporin genes) or acquired (secondary to chronic renal disorders such as polycystic kidney disease), or it may be an adverse effect of lithium therapy.[104,130] Polyuria is compensated by equivalent polydipsia. Similar to central DI, preexisting nephrogenic DI can worsen during pregnancy before improving after delivery.

Treatment of Diabetes Insipidus During Pregnancy

dDAVP is the mainstay therapy for DI during pregnancy, whether it is transient or preexisting, and whether it is unmasked or exacerbated by the pregnancy.[115] Unlike AVP, this analogue of AVP is resistant to vasopressinase.[109,111,128,131]

When preexisting central DI is controlled by dDAVP before conception, treatment can be continued during pregnancy, although an increase in the dose may be necessary.

The few available data on the safety of dDAVP for the mother and unborn child are reassuring.[131,132]

SUMMARY

LH may occur during pregnancy and in the postpartum period, and patients often present with headache, vision problems, and a pituitary deficiency. MRI typically shows a pituitary mass with intense enhancement after gadolinium injection, if it is performed, which may differentiate LH from NFPAs. At present, the condition is diagnosed based on clinical and neuroradiological data, and it does not require a biopsy. The course, in terms of mass effect, is generally spontaneously favorable but it may require the administration of corticosteroids or even transsphenoidal resection. The course of pituitary deficiencies is highly variable; some cases recover over time, whereas others persist indefinitely.

Sheehan syndrome is currently a very rare condition in developed countries, although it continues to be frequently observed in developing countries. It is related to a pituitary infarction secondary to a massive peripartum hemorrhage. It is responsible for agalactia and amenorrhea, which often are neglected, and the diagnosis is thus generally made after a delay of many years. Gonadotropic and somatotropic function are always deficient.

Sellar or parasellar tumors other than pituitary adenomas (craniopharyngiomas, meningiomas, and so forth) may also be detected during pregnancy, and their management may be difficult, particularly regarding the risks associated with surgery to the fetus.

DI is a rare complication of pregnancy. It is related to the increased placental production of vasopressinase, which inactivates circulating vasopressin and is thus usually transient, occurring late in pregnancy and disappearing a few days after delivery. Preexisting central or nephrogenic DI is occasionally unmasked by pregnancy.

REFERENCES

1. Caturegli P, Newschaffer C, Olivi A, et al. Autoimmune hypophysitis. Endocr Rev 2005;26(5):599–614.

2. Gubbi S, Hannah-Shmouni F, Stratakis CA, et al. Primary hypophysitis and other autoimmune disorders of the sellar and suprasellar regions. Rev Endocr Metab Disord 2018;19(4):335–47.
3. Caturegli P, Lupi I, Landek-Salgado M, et al. Pituitary autoimmunity: 30 years later. Autoimmun Rev 2008;7(8):631–7.
4. Falorni A, Minarelli V, Bartoloni E, et al. Diagnosis and classification of autoimmune hypophysitis. Autoimmun Rev 2014;13(4–5):412–6.
5. Joshi MN, Whitelaw BC, Carroll PV. Mechanisms in endocrinology: hypophysitis: diagnosis and treatment. Eur J Endocrinol 2018;179(3):R151–63.
6. Prete A, Salvatori R. Hypophysitis. In: De Groot LJ, Chrousos G, Dungan K, et al, editors. Endotext. South Dartmouth (MA): MDText.com, NCBI Bookshelfpp; 2000. p. 1–26.
7. Fehn M, Sommer C, Ludecke DK, et al. Lymphocytic hypophysitis: light and electron microscopic findings and correlation to clinical appearance. Endocr Pathol 1998;9(1):71–8.
8. Chiloiro S, Tartaglione T, Angelini F, et al. An overview of diagnosis of primary autoimmune hypophysitis in a prospective single-center experience. Neuroendocrinology 2017;104(3):280–90.
9. Honegger J, Schlaffer S, Menzel C, et al. Diagnosis of primary hypophysitis in germany. J Clin Endocrinol Metab 2015;100(10):3841–9.
10. Khare S, Jagtap VS, Budyal SR, et al. Primary (autoimmune) hypophysitis: a single centre experience. Pituitary 2015;18(1):16–22.
11. Wang S, Wang L, Yao Y, et al. Primary lymphocytic hypophysitis: Clinical characteristics and treatment of 50 cases in a single centre in China over 18 years. Clin Endocrinol (Oxf) 2017;87(2):177–84.
12. Gutenberg A, Larsen J, Lupi I, et al. A radiologic score to distinguish autoimmune hypophysitis from nonsecreting pituitary adenoma preoperatively. AJNR Am J Neuroradiol 2009;30(9):1766–72.
13. Goudie RB, Pinkerton PH. Anterior hypophysitis and Hashimoto's disease in a young woman. J Pathol Bacteriol 1962;83:584–5.
14. Guay AT, Agnello V, Tronic BC, et al. Lymphocytic hypophysitis in a man. J Clin Endocrinol Metab 1987;64(3):631–4.
15. Caturegli P, Di Dalmazi G, Lombardi M, et al. Hypophysitis secondary to cytotoxic T-lymphocyte-associated protein 4 blockade: insights into pathogenesis from an autopsy series. Am J Pathol 2016;186(12):3225–35.
16. Honegger J, Giese S. Acute pituitary disease in pregnancy: how to handle hypophysitis and Sheehan's syndrome. Minerva Endocrinol 2018;43(4):465–75.
17. McGrail KM, Beyerl BD, Black PM, et al. Lymphocytic adenohypophysitis of pregnancy with complete recovery. Neurosurgery 1987;20(5):791–3.
18. Stelmach M, O'Day J. Rapid change in visual fields associated with suprasellar lymphocytic hypophysitis. J Clin Neuroophthalmol 1991;11(1):19–24.
19. Nussbaum CE, Okawara SH, Jacobs LS. Lymphocytic hypophysitis with involvement of the cavernous sinus and hypothalamus. Neurosurgery 1991;28(3):440–4.
20. Supler ML, Mickle JP. Lymphocytic hypophysitis: report of a case in a man with cavernous sinus involvement. Surg Neurol 1992;37(6):472–6.
21. Pekic S, Bogosavljevic V, Peker S, et al. Lymphocytic hypophysitis successfully treated with stereotactic radiosurgery: case report and review of the literature. J Neurol Surg A Cent Eur Neurosurg 2018;79(1):77–85.
22. Tubridy N, Molloy J, Saunders D, et al. Postpartum pituitary hypophysitis. J Neuroophthalmol 2001;21(2):106–8.

23. Cortet C, Barat P, Zenaty D, et al. Group 5: acute adrenal insufficiency in adults and pediatric patients. Ann Endocrinol (Paris) 2017;78(6):535–43.

24. Cosman F, Post KD, Holub DA, et al. Lymphocytic hypophysitis. Report of 3 new cases and review of the literature. Medicine (Baltimore) 1989;68(4):240–56.

25. Pressman EK, Zeidman SM, Reddy UM, et al. Differentiating lymphocytic adenohypophysitis from pituitary adenoma in the peripartum patient. J Reprod Med 1995;40(4):251–9.

26. Davies EC, Jakobiec FA, Stagner AM, et al. An atypical case of lymphocytic panhypophysitis in a pregnant woman. J Neuroophthalmol 2016;36(3):313–6.

27. Sakurai K, Yamashita R, Niituma S, et al. Usefulness of anti-rabphilin-3A antibodies for diagnosing central diabetes insipidus in the third trimester of pregnancy. Endocr J 2017;64(6):645–50.

28. Gal R, Schwartz A, Gukovsky-Oren S, et al. Lymphoid hypophysitis associated with sudden maternal death: report of a case review of the literature. Obstet Gynecol Surv 1986;41(10):619–21.

29. Blisard KS, Pfalzgraf RR, Balko MG. Sudden death due to lymphoplasmacytic hypophysitis. Am J Forensic Med Pathol 1992;13(3):207–10.

30. Thodou E, Asa SL, Kontogeorgos G, et al. Clinical case seminar: lymphocytic hypophysitis: clinicopathological findings. J Clin Endocrinol Metab 1995;80(8):2302–11.

31. Angelousi A, Cohen C, Sosa S, et al. Clinical, endocrine and imaging characteristics of patients with primary hypophysitis. Horm Metab Res 2018;50(4):296–302.

32. Arafah BM, Prunty D, Ybarra J, et al. The dominant role of increased intrasellar pressure in the pathogenesis of hypopituitarism, hyperprolactinemia, and headaches in patients with pituitary adenomas. J Clin Endocrinol Metab 2000;85(5):1789–93.

33. Barbesino G, Sluss PM, Caturegli P. Central hypothyroidism in a patient with pituitary autoimmunity: evidence for TSH-independent thyroid hormone synthesis. J Clin Endocrinol Metab 2012;97(2):345–50.

34. Tirosh A, Hirsch D, Robenshtok E, et al. Variations in clinical and imaging findings by time of diagnosis in females with hypopituitarism attributed to lymphocytic hypophysitis. Endocr Pract 2016;22(4):447–53.

35. Gagneja H, Arafah B, Taylor HC. Histologically proven lymphocytic hypophysitis: spontaneous resolution and subsequent pregnancy. Mayo Clin Proc 1999;74(2):150–4.

36. Howlett TA, Levy MJ, Robertson IJ. How reliably can autoimmune hypophysitis be diagnosed without pituitary biopsy. Clin Endocrinol (Oxf) 2010;73(1):18–21.

37. Powrie JK, Powell M, Ayers AB, et al. Lymphocytic adenohypophysitis: magnetic resonance imaging features of two new cases and a review of the literature. Clin Endocrinol (Oxf) 1995;42(3):315–22.

38. Unluhizarci K, Bayram F, Colak R, et al. Distinct radiological and clinical appearance of lymphocytic hypophysitis. J Clin Endocrinol Metab 2001;86(5):1861–4.

39. Fujisawa I. Magnetic resonance imaging of the hypothalamic-neurohypophyseal system. J Neuroendocrinol 2004;16(4):297–302.

40. Fujisawa I, Nishimura K, Asato R, et al. Posterior lobe of the pituitary in diabetes insipidus: MR findings. J Comput Assist Tomogr 1987;11(2):221–5.

41. Liu W, Wang L, Liu M, et al. Pituitary morphology and function in 43 children with central diabetes insipidus. Int J Endocrinol 2016;2016:6365830.

42. Ahmadi J, Meyers GS, Segall HD, et al. Lymphocytic adenohypophysitis: contrast-enhanced MR imaging in five cases. Radiology 1995;195(1):30–4.

43. Bevan JS, Othman S, Lazarus JH, et al. Reversible adrenocorticotropin deficiency due to probable autoimmune hypophysitis in a woman with postpartum thyroiditis. J Clin Endocrinol Metab 1992;74(3):548–52.
44. Hayes FJ, McKenna TJ. The occurrence of lymphocytic hypophysitis in a first but not subsequent pregnancy. J Clin Endocrinol Metab 1996;81(8):3131–2.
45. Ikeda H, Okudaira Y. Spontaneous regression of pituitary mass in temporal association with pregnancy. Neuroradiology 1987;29(5):488–92.
46. Komatsu M, Kondo T, Yamauchi K, et al. Antipituitary antibodies in patients with the primary empty sella syndrome. J Clin Endocrinol Metab 1988;67(4):633–8.
47. Jenkins PJ, Chew SL, Lowe DG, et al. Lymphocytic hypophysitis: unusual features of a rare disorder. Clin Endocrinol (Oxf) 1995;42(5):529–34.
48. Pestell RG, Best JD, Alford FP. Lymphocytic hypophysitis. The clinical spectrum of the disorder and evidence for an autoimmune pathogenesis. Clin Endocrinol (Oxf) 1990;33(4):457–66.
49. Sinha D, Sinha A, Pirie AM. A case of recurrent lymphocytic hypophysitis in pregnancy. J Obstet Gynaecol 2006;26(3):255–6.
50. Husebye ES, Anderson MS, Kampe O. Autoimmune polyendocrine syndromes. N Engl J Med 2018;378(26):2543–4.
51. Crock P, Salvi M, Miller A, et al. Detection of anti-pituitary autoantibodies by immunoblotting. J Immunol Methods 1993;162(1):31–40.
52. Crock PA. Cytosolic autoantigens in lymphocytic hypophysitis. J Clin Endocrinol Metab 1998;83(2):609–18.
53. Hansen BL, Hegedus L, Hansen GN, et al. Pituitary-cell autoantibody diversity in sera from patients with untreated Graves' disease. Autoimmunity 1989;5(1–2):49–57.
54. Nishiki M, Murakami Y, Ozawa Y, et al. Serum antibodies to human pituitary membrane antigens in patients with autoimmune lymphocytic hypophysitis and infundibuloneurohypophysitis. Clin Endocrinol (Oxf) 2001;54(3):327–33.
55. Bellastella G, Maiorino MI, Bizzarro A, et al. Revisitation of autoimmune hypophysitis: knowledge and uncertainties on pathophysiological and clinical aspects. Pituitary 2016;19(6):625–42.
56. Bellastella G, Rotondi M, Pane E, et al. Predictive role of the immunostaining pattern of immunofluorescence and the titers of antipituitary antibodies at presentation for the occurrence of autoimmune hypopituitarism in patients with autoimmune polyendocrine syndromes over a five-year follow-up. J Clin Endocrinol Metab 2010;95(8):3750–7.
57. De Bellis A, Pane E, Bellastella G, et al. Detection of antipituitary and antihypothalamus antibodies to investigate the role of pituitary or hypothalamic autoimmunity in patients with selective idiopathic hypopituitarism. Clin Endocrinol (Oxf) 2011;75(3):361–6.
58. Chanson P, Maiter D. Prolactinoma. In: Melmed S, editor. The pituitary. 4th edition. London: Elsevier; 2017. p. 467–514.
59. Dejager S, Gerber S, Foubert L, et al. Sheehan's syndrome: differential diagnosis in the acute phase. J Intern Med 1998;244(3):261–6.
60. Karaca Z, Kelestimur F. Pregnancy and other pituitary disorders (including GH deficiency). Best Pract Res Clin Endocrinol Metab 2011;25(6):897–910.
61. Karaca Z, Tanriverdi F, Unluhizarci K, et al. Pregnancy and pituitary disorders. Eur J Endocrinol 2010;162(3):453–75.
62. Diri H, Tanriverdi F, Karaca Z, et al. Extensive investigation of 114 patients with Sheehan's syndrome: a continuing disorder. Eur J Endocrinol 2014;171(3):311–8.

63. Bullmann C, Faust M, Hoffmann A, et al. Five cases with central diabetes insipidus and hypogonadism as first presentation of neurosarcoidosis. Eur J Endocrinol 2000;142(4):365–72.
64. Hayashi H, Yamada K, Kuroki T, et al. Lymphocytic hypophysitis and pulmonary sarcoidosis. Report of a case. Am J Clin Pathol 1991;95(4):506–11.
65. Kaltsas GA, Powles TB, Evanson J, et al. Hypothalamo-pituitary abnormalities in adult patients with langerhans cell histiocytosis: clinical, endocrinological, and radiological features and response to treatment. J Clin Endocrinol Metab 2000;85(4):1370–6.
66. de Bruin WI, van't Verlaat JW, Graamans K, et al. Sellar granulomatous mass in a pregnant woman with active Crohn's disease. Neth J Med 1991;39(3–4):136–41.
67. Joneja U, Hooper DC, Evans JJ, et al. Postpartum granulomatous hypophysitis: a case study, review of the literature, and discussion of pathogenesis. Case Rep Pathol 2016;2016:7510323.
68. Fleseriu M, Hashim IA, Karavitaki N, et al. Hormonal replacement in hypopituitarism in adults: an endocrine society clinical practice guideline. J Clin Endocrinol Metab 2016;101(11):3888–921.
69. Biswas M, Thackare H, Jones MK, et al. Lymphocytic hypophysitis and headache in pregnancy. BJOG 2002;109(10):1184–6.
70. Patel MC, Guneratne N, Haq N, et al. Peripartum hypopituitarism and lymphocytic hypophysitis. QJM 1995;88(8):571–80.
71. Ray DK, Yen CP, Vance ML, et al. Gamma knife surgery for lymphocytic hypophysitis. J Neurosurg 2010;112(1):118–21.
72. Broekman M, Goedee SH, Nieuwlaat WA, et al. Corticosteroid treatment buys time in case of a newly diagnosed hypophysitis with visual deterioration. BMJ Case Rep 2013;2013 [pii:bcr2013010035].
73. Reusch JE, Kleinschmidt-DeMasters BK, Lillehei KO, et al. Preoperative diagnosis of lymphocytic hypophysitis (adenohypophysitis) unresponsive to short course dexamethasone: case report. Neurosurgery 1992;30(2):268–72.
74. Fujimaki T, Hotta S, Mochizuki T, et al. Pituitary apoplexy as a consequence of lymphocytic adenohypophysitis in a pregnant woman: a case report. Neurol Res 2005;27(4):399–402.
75. McDermott MW, Griesdale DE, Berry K, et al. Lymphocytic adenohypophysitis. Can J Neurol Sci 1988;15(1):38–43.
76. Ramiandrasoa C, Castinetti F, Raingeard I, et al. Delayed diagnosis of Sheehan's syndrome in a developed country: a retrospective cohort study. Eur J Endocrinol 2013;169(4):431–8.
77. Zargar AH, Singh B, Laway BA, et al. Epidemiologic aspects of postpartum pituitary hypofunction (Sheehan's syndrome). Fertil Steril 2005;84(2):523–8.
78. Du GL, Liu ZH, Chen M, et al. Sheehan's syndrome in Xinjiang: Clinical characteristics and laboratory evaluation of 97 patients. Hormones (Athens) 2015; 14(4):660–7.
79. Feinberg EC, Molitch ME, Endres LK, et al. The incidence of Sheehan's syndrome after obstetric hemorrhage. Fertil Steril 2005;84(4):975–9.
80. Higham CE, Johannsson G, Shalet SM. Hypopituitarism. Lancet 2016; 388(10058):2403–15.
81. Atmaca H, Tanriverdi F, Gokce C, et al. Posterior pituitary function in Sheehan's syndrome. Eur J Endocrinol 2007;156(5):563–7.
82. Hayashi M, Tomobe K, Hoshimoto K, et al. Successful pregnancy following gonadotropin therapy in a patient with hypogonadotropic hypogonadism resulting from craniopharyngioma. Int J Clin Pract 2002;56(2):149–51.

83. Sachs BP, Smith SK, Cassar J, et al. Rapid enlargement of carniopharyngioma in pregnancy. Br J Obstet Gynaecol 1978;85(7):577–8.

84. Johnson RJ Jr, Voorhies RM, Witkin M, et al. Fertility following excision of a symptomatic craniopharyngioma during pregnancy: case report. Surg Neurol 1993;39(4):257–62.

85. Hiett AK, Barton JR. Diabetes insipidus associated with craniopharyngioma in pregnancy. Obstet Gynecol 1990;76(5 Pt 2):982–4.

86. van der Wildt B, Drayer JI, Eskes TK. Diabetes insipidus in pregnancy as a first sign of a craniopharyngioma. Eur J Obstet Gynecol Reprod Biol 1980;10(4): 269–74.

87. Maniker AH, Krieger AJ. Rapid recurrence of craniopharyngioma during pregnancy with recovery of vision: a case report. Surg Neurol 1996;45(4):324–7.

88. Magge SN, Brunt M, Scott RM. Craniopharyngioma presenting during pregnancy 4 years after a normal magnetic resonance imaging scan: case report. Neurosurgery 2001;49(4):1014–6 [conclusion: 1016–7].

89. Aydin Y, Can SM, Gulkilik A, et al. Rapid enlargement and recurrence of a preexisting intrasellar craniopharyngioma during the course of two pregnancies. Case report. J Neurosurg 1999;91(2):322–4.

90. Zoia C, Cattalani A, Turpini E, et al. Haemorrhagic presentation of a craniopharyngioma in a pregnant woman. Case Rep Neurol Med 2014;2014:435208.

91. Grillo-Mallo E, Jimenez-Benito J, Diez-Feijoo E, et al. Acute visual loss in pregnancy caused by craniopharyngioma. Arch Soc Esp Oftalmol 2014;89(4):152–6 [in Spanish].

92. Cohen-Gadol AA, Friedman JA, Friedman JD, et al. Neurosurgical management of intracranial lesions in the pregnant patient: a 36-year institutional experience and review of the literature. J Neurosurg 2009;111(6):1150–7.

93. Haas JF, Janisch W, Staneczek W. Newly diagnosed primary intracranial neoplasms in pregnant women: a population-based assessment. J Neurol Neurosurg Psychiatry 1986;49(8):874–80.

94. Laviv Y, Ohla V, Kasper EM. Unique features of pregnancy-related meningiomas: lessons learned from 148 reported cases and theoretical implications of a prolactin modulated pathogenesis. Neurosurg Rev 2018;41(1):95–108.

95. Laviv Y, Bayoumi A, Mahadevan A, et al. Meningiomas in pregnancy: timing of surgery and clinical outcomes as observed in 104 cases and establishment of a best management strategy. Acta Neurochir (Wien) 2018;160(8):1521–9.

96. Lusis EA, Scheithauer BW, Yachnis AT, et al. Meningiomas in pregnancy: a clinicopathologic study of 17 cases. Neurosurgery 2012;71(5):951–61.

97. Hsu DW, Efird JT, Hedley-Whyte ET. Progesterone and estrogen receptors in meningiomas: prognostic considerations. J Neurosurg 1997;86(1):113–20.

98. Perry A, Cai DX, Scheithauer BW, et al. Merlin, DAL-1, and progesterone receptor expression in clinicopathologic subsets of meningioma: a correlative immunohistochemical study of 175 cases. J Neuropathol Exp Neurol 2000;59(10): 872–9.

99. Priddy BH, Otto BA, Carrau RL, et al. Management of skull base tumors in the obstetric population: a case series. World Neurosurg 2018;113:e373–82.

100. Kuczkowski KM. Nonobstetric surgery during pregnancy: what are the risks of anesthesia? Obstet Gynecol Surv 2004;59(1):52–6.

101. Hime MC, Richardson JA. Diabetes insipidus and pregnancy. Case report, incidence and review of literature. Obstet Gynecol Surv 1978;33(6):375–9.

102. Moore K, Thompson C, Trainer P. Disorders of water balance. Clin Med 2003; 3(1):28–33.

103. Bichet DG. The posterior pituitary. In: Melmed S, editor. The pituitary. 3rd edition. Malden (MA): Blackwell Science; 2011. p. 261–99.

104. Bichet DG. Diabètes insipides. In: Chanson P, Young J, editors. Traité d'Endocrinologie. Paris: Flammarion Médecine-Sciences; 2007. p. 995–1013.

105. Schneider HJ, Aimaretti G, Kreitschmann-Andermahr I, et al. Hypopituitarism. Lancet 2007;369(9571):1461–70.

106. Fenske W, Allolio B. Clinical review: current state and future perspectives in the diagnosis of diabetes insipidus: a clinical review. J Clin Endocrinol Metab 2012; 97(10):3426–37.

107. Ananthakrishnan S. Diabetes insipidus in pregnancy: etiology, evaluation, and management. Endocr Pract 2009;15(4):377–82.

108. Qureshi S, Galiveeti S, Bichet DG, et al. Diabetes insipidus: celebrating a century of vasopressin therapy. Endocrinology 2014;155(12):4605–21.

109. Barron WM, Cohen LH, Ulland LA, et al. Transient vasopressin-resistant diabetes insipidus of pregnancy. N Engl J Med 1984;310(7):442–4.

110. Davison JM, Sheills EA, Barron WM, et al. Changes in the metabolic clearance of vasopressin and in plasma vasopressinase throughout human pregnancy. J Clin Invest 1989;83(4):1313–8.

111. Davison JM, Sheills EA, Philips PR, et al. Metabolic clearance of vasopressin and an analogue resistant to vasopressinase in human pregnancy. Am J Physiol 1993;264(2 Pt 2):F348–53.

112. Lindheimer MD, Davison JM. Osmoregulation, the secretion of arginine vasopressin and its metabolism during pregnancy. Eur J Endocrinol 1995;132(2): 133–43.

113. Barron WM, Durr J, Stamoutsos BA, et al. Osmoregulation and vasopressin secretion during pregnancy in Brattleboro rats. Am J Physiol 1985;248(1 Pt 2): R29–37.

114. Schrier RW. Systemic arterial vasodilation, vasopressin, and vasopressinase in pregnancy. J Am Soc Nephrol 2010;21(4):570–2.

115. Chanson P, Salenave S. Diabetes insipidus and pregnancy. Ann Endocrinol (Paris) 2016;77(2):135–8.

116. Christ-Crain M, Fenske W. Copeptin in the diagnosis of vasopressin-dependent disorders of fluid homeostasis. Nat Rev Endocrinol 2016;12(3):168–76.

117. Kollamparambil TG, Mohan PV, Gunasuntharam K, et al. Prenatal presentation of transient central diabetes insipidus. Eur J Pediatr 2011;170(5):653–6.

118. Weinberg LE, Dinsmoor MJ, Silver RK. Severe hydramnios and preterm delivery in association with transient maternal diabetes insipidus. Obstet Gynecol 2010; 116(Suppl 2):547–9.

119. Sainz Bueno JA, Villarejo Ortiz P, Hidalgo Amat J, et al. Transient diabetes insipidus during pregnancy: a clinical case and a review of the syndrome. Eur J Obstet Gynecol Reprod Biol 2005;118(2):251–4.

120. Durr JA, Hoggard JG, Hunt JM, et al. Diabetes insipidus in pregnancy associated with abnormally high circulating vasopressinase activity. N Engl J Med 1987;316(17):1070–4.

121. Durr JA. Diabetes insipidus in pregnancy. Am J Kidney Dis 1987;9(4):276–83.

122. Katz VL, Bowes WA Jr. Transient diabetes insipidus and preeclampsia. South Med J 1987;80(4):524–5.

123. Kennedy S, Hall PM, Seymour AE, et al. Transient diabetes insipidus and acute fatty liver of pregnancy. Br J Obstet Gynaecol 1994;101(5):387–91.

124. Brewster UC, Hayslett JP. Diabetes insipidus in the third trimester of pregnancy. Obstet Gynecol 2005;105(5 Pt 2):1173–6.

125. Durr JA, Lindheimer MD. Diagnosis and management of diabetes insipidus during pregnancy. Endocr Pract 1996;2(5):353–61.
126. Yamanaka Y, Takeuchi K, Konda E, et al. Transient postpartum diabetes insipidus in twin pregnancy associated with HELLP syndrome. J Perinat Med 2002; 30(3):273–5.
127. Woelk JL, Dombroski RA, Brezina PR. Gestational diabetes insipidus, HELLP syndrome and eclampsia in a twin pregnancy: a case report. J Perinatol 2010;30(2):144–5.
128. Wallia A, Bizhanova A, Huang W, et al. Acute diabetes insipidus mediated by vasopressinase after placental abruption. J Clin Endocrinol Metab 2013;98(3): 881–6.
129. Iwasaki Y, Oiso Y, Kondo K, et al. Aggravation of subclinical diabetes insipidus during pregnancy. N Engl J Med 1991;324(8):522–6.
130. Bockenhauer D, Bichet DG. Pathophysiology, diagnosis and management of nephrogenic diabetes insipidus. Nat Rev Nephrol 2015;11(10):576–88.
131. Kallen BA, Carlsson SS, Bengtsson BK. Diabetes insipidus and use of desmopressin (Minirin) during pregnancy. Eur J Endocrinol 1995;132(2):144–6.
132. Ray JG. DDAVP use during pregnancy: an analysis of its safety for mother and child. Obstet Gynecol Surv 1998;53(7):450–5.

Pheochromocytoma and Pregnancy

Jacques W.M. Lenders, MD, PhD[a,b,]*, Katharina Langton, MSc[c],
Johan F. Langenhuijsen, MD, PhD[d], Graeme Eisenhofer, PhD[b,c]

KEYWORDS

- Pheochromocytoma • Paraganglioma • Pregnancy • Catecholamines
- Metanephrines

KEY POINTS

- Timely consideration of a pheochromocytoma or paraganglioma before or in pregnancy is key for achieving optimal outcome for mother and fetus.
- For biochemical testing, measurements plasma or urinary free metanephrines are tests of first choice as in nonpregnant patients.
- For locating a pheochromocytoma or paraganglioma, MRI is *first choice* in pregnancy; all functional imaging is contraindicated.
- Tumor removal before 24 weeks of gestation, during cesarean delivery, or postpartum provides the best outcome.

INTRODUCTION

Neuroendocrine chromaffin cell tumors comprise pheochromocytomas and paragangliomas (PPGLs), which arise from chromaffin cells of the adrenal medulla (80%–85%) and are associated with the sympathetic ganglia (15%–20%), respectively.[1] Prevalence depends on disease presentation, varying from low in patients with hypertension (0.2%–0.6%) to high in patients with an incidentally discovered adrenal mass (3%–7%).[2–4] Despite the availability of accurate diagnostic tests, the prevalence of

Disclosure: The authors do not have any relationship with any public, commercial, or not-for-profit organization regarding this article.
[a] Department of Internal Medicine, Radboud University Medical Center, Geert Grooteplein Zuid 8, 6525 GA Nijmegen, The Netherlands; [b] Department of Medicine III, Carl Gustav Carus University Medical Centre, Dresden, Germany; [c] Institute of Clinical Chemistry and Laboratory Medicine, Medical Faculty Carl Gustav Carus, Technische Universität Dresden, Fetcherstrasse 74, 01307 Dresden, Germany; [d] Department of Urology, Radboud University Medical Centre, Geert Grooteplein Zuid 10, 6525 GA Nijmegen, The Netherlands
* Corresponding author. Department of Internal Medicine, Radboud University Medical Center, Geert Grooteplein Zuid 8, 6525 GA Nijmegen, the Netherlands.
E-mail address: jacques.lenders@radboudumc.nl

Endocrinol Metab Clin N Am 48 (2019) 605–617
https://doi.org/10.1016/j.ecl.2019.05.006   endo.theclinics.com

undiagnosed PPGLs in autopsy studies is considerable (0.05%–0.1%).[5] Missing the tumor during life is attributed to not considering the possibility of the tumor, because of the aspecific nature of the signs and symptoms associated with the production of catecholamines. Nevertheless, the excess production of catecholamines is responsible for a variety of paroxysmal symptoms such as palpitations, sweating, and headache. More importantly, the strong surges of catecholamine secretion are responsible for the increased risk of cardiovascular morbidity and mortality.[6–8] PPGLs may be part of several hereditary syndromes. Up to 40% of all patients with a PPGL have a pathogenic germline mutation.[9] Because pregnant patients are relatively young, the proportion of pregnant patients with PPGL who have an underlying mutation in one of the PPGL susceptibility genes might be even higher.

The prevalence of PPGL, being low in hypertensive patients, is even lower in patients who have hypertension and are pregnant. The occurrence of a PPGL during pregnancy has been estimated as 1 in 15,000 to 54,000 pregnancies.[10–12] Although this is an extremely rare combination, the occurrence of a PPGL during pregnancy may result in serious and even fatal cardiovascular complications in mother and fetus.[13] The ultimate outcome is predominantly dependent on whether the diagnosis is missed antepartum or not.

Studies before 1970 described high respective maternal and fetal mortalities of 48% and 54% if the diagnosis was missed antenatally, whereas other studies showed substantially lower respective mortalities of less than 5% and less than 15%, if the diagnosis was made antenally.[10,14–17] The latter findings were supported by a systematic review comprising 135 case reports, showing respective maternal and fetal mortalities of 8% and 17%.[18] More telling was the finding that all mothers in whom the diagnosis was made antenatally survived, compared with only 71% of those in whom the diagnosis missed antenatally. Another recent systematic review suggested that the outcome of women with a paraganglioma may be better than with a pheochromocytoma.[19] It is unknown whether differences in outcome are related to differences in biochemical phenotype. The awareness of caregivers of the beneficial effects of diagnosing and treating a PPGL antenatally has led to an increase in the proportion of patients in whom an antenatal diagnosis was made, although this has plateaued over the last decades to between 70% and 75%.[18] This implies that a considerable number of patients with the tumor are still missed before delivery.

A major reason why the diagnosis of a PPGL is not considered in a timely manner during pregnancy is the misconception that hypertension in pregnancy cannot be anything else other than gestational hypertension or (pre)eclampsia. Indeed, pregnancy-associated hypertension is much more prevalent than a PPGL, but in view of the potential devastating consequences of missing a PPGL in pregnancy, a low threshold of suspicion is warranted. It is therefore pivotal that caregivers of pregnant women such as midwives and obstetricians should be aware of the clinical clues that might point to a PPGL. Today biochemical exclusion or confirmation of this tumor is much less complex than in the past. Finally, once a PPGL has been confirmed the best outcome is ensured if patients are managed by a multidisciplinary team and this pertains a fortiori to pregnant patients with a PPGL.[4]

In this review we will address the following questions: What are the effects of catecholamines in pregnancy in a woman with a PPGL? What are the clinical clues that should alarm caregivers about the potential presence of a PPGL? How to establish the diagnosis of a PPGL in a pregnant patient? What is the best time to remove the tumor and how to prepare the patient for surgery? Finally, the preferred mode of delivery in a patient harboring a PPGL is addressed.

WHAT ARE THE EFFECTS OF CATECHOLAMINES IN PREGNANCY IN A WOMAN WITH PHEOCHROMOCYTOMA OR PARAGANGLIOMA?

Catecholamines, including norepinephrine, epinephrine and dopamine, are potent cardio- and vasoactive compounds with numerous physiologic functions, even beyond cardiovascular homeostasis. Norepinephrine is a major neurotransmitter of the sympathetic nervous system, whereas epinephrine is a hormone near exclusively produced by the adrenal medulla. Both catecholamines play a central role in the adaptation to and protection against stressful stimuli, including pregnancy and birth. In healthy pregnant women, plasma and urinary catecholamine levels are not consistently increased.[20–22] Even in preeclampsia where an increased sympathetic activity is suggested to play some pathophysiologic role, maternal plasma catecholamine levels are only slightly increased.[23] It has been suggested that patients with eclampsia might have increased plasma catecholamine levels at the time of admission for an eclamptic fit that then return to normal within a few days.[24]

Maternal catecholamines hardly cross the placental barrier and even in patients harboring a PPGL the umbilical cord blood contains less than 10% of the maternal catecholamine concentrations.[25,26] The placenta plays a key role in protection of the fetus against exposure to high catecholamine levels coming from the tumor. This is due to the presence of norepinephrine transporters and catecholamine metabolizing enzymes (such as monoamine-oxidase and catechol-O-methyltransferase) in the placenta.[25,27] These transporters facilitate norepinephrine uptake, whereas the enzymes terminate the biological activity of the catecholamines. Although the fetus itself has a high secretion rate of catecholamines, an extremely effective clearance results in low circulating levels of catecholamines.[28] Levels of catecholamines are particularly high during delivery to assist the fetus in the stressful passage through the birth canal and to adapt to early postnatal life.[29]

Patients with a PPGL may have sustained hypertension, paroxysmal hypertension, or hypertensive paroxysms on top of sustained hypertension.[1] Sustained hypertension in pregnancy is associated with adverse effects such as intrauterine growth retardation, superimposed preeclampsia, and perinatal death.[30] In patients with a catecholamine-producing tumor such as a PPGL, circulating catecholamines in the mother can rise to extremely high levels, which may jeopardize critically the function of many organs, including the placenta. Such ephemeral spiking levels of catecholamines in the mother during pregnancy may have severe deleterious effects on the uteroplacental circulation.[31] The major effect is strong intermittent vasoconstriction in this specific and vulnerable vascular bed, resulting in increased fetal mortality due to placental abruption and intrauterine hypoxia.

WHICH CLINICAL CLUES SHOULD ALARM CAREGIVERS OF THE POTENTIAL PRESENCE OF PHEOCHROMOCYTOMA OR PARAGANGLIOMA?

There are several relevant clinical clues that should alarm obstetricians and midwives immediately to think of a PPGL. This requires a thorough medical history (including recent medication) and physical examination. The most straightforward clues in a pregnant patient with hypertension can be derived from the previous history and family history. Patients with a previous PPGL or who are carriers of one of the susceptibility genes are at an increased risk to develop a recurrence or a first PPGL. Nearly 40% of all patients with a PPGL have a pathogenic germline mutation and usually these patients present at younger age and have a higher risk of multifocal, recurrent, and metastatic disease. The most well-known mutated genes include *RET* (*rearranged during transfection*), *VHL* (*von Hippel-Lindau*), *NF1* (*neurofibromatosis I*), *SDH* (*succinate* dehydrogenase subunits *SDHA, SDHB, SDHC, SDHD), FH (fumarate hydratase),* *TMEM127 (transmembrane domain protein 127),* and *MAX (MYC-associated factor X).*[9,32] One should therefore be aware that the specific features of the associated hereditary PPGLs syndromes may help in a timely consideration of a PPGL. This applies in particular to the MEN2 (multiple endocrine neoplasia type 2), NF1, VHL, and the familial paraganglioma syndromes syndromes (PGL 1–5) (**Table 1**).

The clinical presentation of a PPGL during pregnancy is not essentially different from that in nonpregnant patients. Signs or symptoms can vary from minor to typical paroxysmal symptoms (such as headache, sweating, hypertension, and palpitations) or to severe life-threatening cardiovascular complications or even multiorgan failure. Most patients may become progressively symptomatic along the time of gestation.[14] This may be explained by mechanical factors such as the growing uterus, fetal movements, uterine contractions, abdominal palpation, and pharmacologic factors such anesthesia.[33] These factors may also be even responsible for a sudden precipitation of a hypertensive PPGL crisis, sometimes evolving into a life-threatening catastrophe such as an acute coronary syndrome, cardiomyopathy, arrhythmias, stroke, syncope, and shock.[34] More rarely a patient may present with noncardiac pulmonary edema, aortic dissection, or unexplained peripartum cardiomyopathy. When a pregnant woman presents with one of these serious acute cardiovascular emergencies, even without known hypertension, one should be aware of a potential underlying PPGL. It is not surprising that the highest risk of these dangerous emergencies is associated with the peripartum period. From larger series in the literature it is clear that nearly

Table 1
The major hereditary syndromes of pheochromocytoma and/or paraganglioma and associated syndromic features

Hereditary Syndromes	Affected Genes	Associated Syndromic Features Other than Pheochromocytoma or Paraganglioma
Multiple endocrine neoplasia type 2A (MEN-2A)	*RET gene*	Primary hyperparathyroidism Medullary thyroid cancer Cutaneous lichen amyloidosis
von Hippel-Lindau syndrome (VHL)	*VHL gene*	Hemangioblastoma of the central nervous system Retinal angioma Renal cell carcinoma Pancreatic neuroendocrine tumor or adenoma Endolymphatic sac tumor of the middle ear Cystadenoma of the epididymis and broad ligament
Neurofibromatosis type I (NF1)	*NF1 gene*	Neurofibromas in skin Axillary and inguinal freckling Iris hamartoma (Lisch nodules) Bone abnormalities Glioma in the central nervous system
Familial paraganglioma syndromes (PGL 1–5)	PGL 1: *SDHD* PGL 2: *SDHAF2* PGL 3: *SDHC* PGL 4: *SDHB* PGL 5: *SDHA*	Gastric stroma tumor (SDHA, B, C, D) Pituitary adenoma (SDHA, B, C, D) Renal cell carcinoma (SDHA, B, D)

90% of the patients report 1 or more symptoms antenatally, yet the diagnosis at that stage is only made in 73% of the patients.[18,35] This implies that the diagnosis is made postdelivery or even postmortem in nearly 3 out of every 10 patients.

There are a few important symptoms that are notorious for confusing clinicians and midwives, resulting in ignoring the potential presence of a PPGL. The most relevant one is hypertension. The prevalence of hypertension in pregnancy is 3% to 5% but is probably higher in obstetric clinics.[36] It is however also a prominent feature of a PPGL.[1] There are significant clinical differences between pregnancy-related and PPGL-related hypertension that may help in differentiating whether there is just pregnancy-related hypertension or hypertension due to a PPGL (**Table 2**).[33] Hypertension in the context of a PPGL can develop in any phase of pregnancy, whereas preeclampsia is limited to the last 20 weeks of pregnancy. Furthermore, PPGL-related paroxysmal hypertension is uncommon for gestational hypertension or preeclampsia. PPGL-related hypertension is generally not associated with ankle edema, proteinuria, or an increased plasma uric acid level; these features are well compatible with gestational hypertension or preeclampsia. A specific symptom that should arouse immediate suspicion of a PPGL is orthostatic hypotension in a pregnant hypertensive woman. In general orthostatic hypotension rules out pregnancy-related hypertension if a simple explanation for this sign is lacking. Nausea can occur in both pregnancy-related hypertension and PPGL and therefore the presence or absence of this symptom does not argue against either diagnosis.

HOW TO ESTABLISH THE DIAGNOSIS OF PHEOCHROMOCYTOMA OR PARAGANGLIOMA IN A PREGNANT PATIENT?

Once there is any clinical suspicion that a pregnant hypertensive patient might have a PPGL, proper biochemical testing is the first step to rule out or confirm this diagnosis.[4] Biochemical testing for a PPGL in pregnant patients is not essentially different from nonpregnant patients, although there are no clinical studies that have assessed the accuracy of biochemical tests or established specific reference values in a pregnant population.

A first consideration when ordering a biochemical test is the question which drugs the patient is using, as they can interfere with the test results. Interference depends largely on the type of assay that is used but nowadays, with the availability of sensitive and specific assays such as LC-MS/MS (liquid chromatography-tandem mass spectrometry), it is mainly pharmacodynamic drug interference that should be considered.[4]

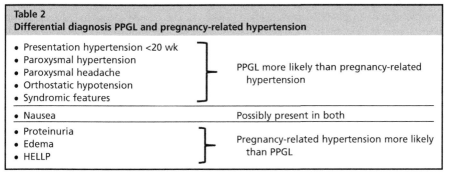

Table 2
Differential diagnosis PPGL and pregnancy-related hypertension

• Presentation hypertension <20 wk • Paroxysmal hypertension • Paroxysmal headache • Orthostatic hypotension • Syndromic features	PPGL more likely than pregnancy-related hypertension
• Nausea	Possibly present in both
• Proteinuria • Edema • HELLP	Pregnancy-related hypertension more likely than PPGL

Abbreviations: HELLP: hemolysis, increased liver enzymes, low platelets; PPGL: pheochromocytoma or paraganglioma.

Antihypertensive drugs, frequently used in pregnancy such as α-methyldopa and labetalol, may be a source of analytical interference in some LC-electrochemical detection assays but not in LC-MS/MS assays. Drugs well known to cause pharmacodynamic interference are tricyclic antidepressants because they interfere with neuronal norepinephrine uptake, thus resulting in false-positive test results.

For the biochemical diagnosis several tests are available with LC-MS/MS as the most accurate method of analysis.[37] For initial screening it was recommended to measure the O-methylated metabolites of catecholamines, metanephrines, either in plasma or urine.[4] A more recent study demonstrated that measurements of the plasma and urinary free metabolites (metanephrines and 3-methoxytyramine) show similar diagnostic performance in patients with low a priori risk, whereas the plasma test is superior to the urine test in patients with a high a priori risk for a PPGL.[38] The high diagnostic sensitivity of the plasma free metabolites (97.9%) with the associated nearly maximal negative predictive value implicates that a PPGL can be considered as excluded if the plasma free metabolites are within the normal range. Exceptions include patients with small or completely nonfunctional tumors (ie, those that do not synthesize catecholamines) but are irrelevant for the pregnant patient presenting with signs and symptoms of catecholamine excess. The specificity of both plasma and urinary free metabolites are similar. Both provide the advantages of less false-positive test results compared with commonly measured urinary deconjugated metabolites.

The underlying basis for the excellent diagnostic performance of plasma free metanephrines is that these metabolites are produced within the tumor and diffuse continuously into the circulation.[39] This contrasts with the episodic and variable exocytic release of the parent catecholamines from the tumor into the circulation.

In daily routine clinical care without consideration of appropriate preanalytics 20% to 25% of patients may show false-positive test results for plasma metabolites.[40] Apart from interfering effects of some drugs, an important source of false-positive test results is inappropriate sampling in the sitting instead of recommended supine position. Drawing blood samples in the sitting position without preceding rest results on average in 30% higher plasma normetanephrine values compared with sampling after at least 20 minutes of supine rest.[41] To minimize the number of false-positive results, it is critical to draw a blood sample for the plasma metabolites after at least 20 minutes of supine rest.[42] At some medical centers blood sampling after supine rest is not possible or is regarded as too cumbersome and impractical. For these centers, measurement of urinary metanephrines (preferably free metanephrines) provides the preferred alternative to blood sampling in the sitting position.

Even after applying optimal blood sampling conditions and having excluded interfering effects of drugs, false-positive test results remain possible, due to unrecognized sympathetic activation. In such cases a clonidine suppression test is useful to differentiate false-from true-positive test results.[43] In pregnant patients this test is, however, contraindicated because of potential unacceptable adverse effects for the fetus.

After having obtained clear and unequivocal biochemical evidence that there must be a catecholamine-producing tumor, the tumor needs to be localized by imaging studies. In nonpregnant patients a 2-step procedure is commonly used: first anatomic imaging (computed tomography [CT] scans with and without contrast), followed by functional imaging (eg, ^{123}I-metaiodobenzylguanidine [MIBG]). This diagnostic approach involves, however, radiation exposure and can therefore not be applied in pregnant women. Some clinicians prefer to start anatomic imaging with abdominal ultrasonography as that is routinely done for obstetric reasons. Although it is a widely available, rapid, and cheap procedure, for the diagnosis of a PPGL the diagnostic sensitivity is limited because small tumors can be easily missed, in particular in the third trimester.[44] Therefore, to exclude or to detect a small abdominal or pelvic PPGL, the preferred imaging test in pregnant women is MRI.[4] MRI is considered to be safe during pregnancy.[45] As solid evidence for safety of gadolinium in pregnancy is lacking, it has been recommended to avoid use of gadolinium during pregnancy unless benefits outweigh the potential risks.[46] Even though the spatial resolution of MRI for abdominal tumors is inferior to that of CT scanning, the diagnostic sensitivity of MRI is more or less similar to that of CT scanning (90%–100%). Specificity of MRI is limited (70%–80%) and therefore functional imaging with, for example, MIBG scanning could be complementary to proof that the tumor is indeed a PPGL. These small radioactive compounds may pass the placenta, and therefore functional imaging using radioactive ligands is contraindicated in pregnant women. Finally, obtaining a tissue specimen by tumor biopsy is contraindicated because of the risk of eliciting a hypertensive crisis.[47]

Once the diagnosis of a PPGL is confirmed, all patients should have access to genetic counseling to establish a decision for genetic testing.[4] There are 2 main reasons for genetic testing: (1) identification of patients with specific mutations who have an increased risk of multifocal, recurrent or metastatic disease and who may benefit from personalized follow-up and (2) establishment of an earlier diagnosis and treatment of PPGLs and other syndromic manifestations in relatives of the proband who may also be willing to undergo genetic testing.

WHAT IS THE BEST TIME TO REMOVE THE TUMOR AND HOW TO PREPARE THE PATIENT FOR SURGERY?

One of the most pressing questions for the clinician is what is the best time to remove the PPGL in a pregnant patient? Although some global conclusions can be drawn from the available studies, we have to realize that the data come from small retrospective studies with the inherent risks of bias. In addition, it is not always possible to dissect the cause of negative outcome: is it due to PPGL per se or to the installed treatment? Surgical removal of the tumor may jeopardize the pregnancy and it is therefore critical to schedule the optimal time of surgery, that is, resulting in the best outcome for mother and fetus.

Based on available studies that have addressed this question, it can be recommended to remove the tumor either before 24 weeks of gestation or at or after delivery. A recent systematic review has shown that in 18 of 56 patients in whom the tumor was removed antenatally, resulted in a full successful outcome in all mothers and fetuses.[18] Before 24 weeks of gestation, the risk of spontaneous abortion is lowest in the second trimester. In the third trimester, anatomic conditions are less favorable for surgical tumor removal. Therefore, in those patients in whom the PPGL is diagnosed in the last trimester, it is preferred to commence medical treatment to protect the mother for catecholamine excess (see next paragraph) and to defer tumor removal until the fetus is viable, so until or after delivery. As this drug regimen is similar to that used for presurgical preparation of tumor removal, some centers choose for one combined surgical session of cesarean delivery and tumor removal.[18] The alternative strategy is to postpone surgery for several weeks after delivery. This has the potential advantage of allowing for functional imaging.

The treatment of first choice in pregnant women is laparoscopic tumor removal.[18] A transperitoneal approach, with the patient in the lateral decubitus position, is usually preferred over any other approach, as this is the most widely used technique in laparoscopic adrenal surgery because of the large working space, especially in the pregnant patient. Theoretically, a retroperitoneal approach in the lateral decubitus position could be favorable to the mother and the fetus, because less use of narcotics leading to fetal depression is needed, shorter operating time and a fast recovery of peristalsis and rapid return to normal diet is expected. This may be less stressful to the mother and fetus than in any other approach. In general, CO_2 insufflation into the small retroperitoneal compartment may lead to less hemodynamic instability than during transperitoneal laparoscopy. However, no comparative surgical studies are available. A posterior retroperitoneal approach should be avoided, as the prone position of the pregnant patient can lead to decreased venous return because of pressure of the enlarged uterus on the inferior caval vein. Diminished venous return also applies to pregnant patients in the lateral decubitus position, especially in the right lateral decubitus position for left-sided adrenalectomy, with an ensuing risk of uteroplacental hypoperfusion. By using the anterior tilt combined with reverse Trendelenburg positioning of the patient, the venous return is improved by releasing the pressure of the uterus on the caval vein. In any laparoscopic approach the introduction of the first trocart should be by open technique to avoid damage to the uterus, pneumoperitoneal pressure should be minimized and not exceed 15 mm Hg (in retroperitoneal surgery not above 20 mm Hg), a constant monitoring is advised of both the uterine and fetal status, as well as maternal CO_2 and arterial blood gases.[48]

In nonpregnant patients the laparoscopic adrenalectomy has been shown to result in less intraoperative hemodynamic instability, shorter hospital stay, and less morbidity than open surgery.[49] In a small series of 14 pregnant women who underwent surgery in the second trimester, 8 underwent laparoscopic adrenalectomy with excellent results.[18] Follow-up at 2 to 6 weeks after surgery is required in all patients to ascertain complete tumor removal by measurements of plasma or urine metanephrines.[50] Long-term annual follow-up after surgery is mandatory in all patients for at least 10 years and should include measurements of blood pressure and plasma or urinary metanephrines. Thereafter, annual follow-up should be continued lifelong only in young patients, those with a germline mutation, and those with an extra-adrenal or large tumor, as they have an increased risk for recurrent disease.[50]

A proper multidisciplinary presurgical preparation is mandatory in all patients with a PPGL but this applies in particular to pregnant patients because, in addition to the mother, a vulnerable fetus is involved. In general, perioperative mortality of PPGL surgery has decreased in the last decades to less than 1%, but there are no reliable data available specifically for the pregnant population. Proper presurgical preparation of patients and tremendous progress in anesthesiology have critically contributed to this achievement.

The first and foremost aim of medical preparation is to minimize the risk of serious complications due to massive release of catecholamines during surgical resection and manipulation of tumors. The mainstay of adequate presurgical preparation of patients with a PPGL, also in pregnant women, is α-adrenoceptor blockade. This advice is not based on randomized clinical trials. Nevertheless, it has been shown in a retrospective study that pregnant women who are pretreated by α-adrenoceptor blockade had substantial lower maternal and fetal mortality than those who did not receive α-adrenoceptor blockade.[51] There are no data establishing the preferred α-adrenoceptor blocker or optimal duration of preoperative treatment.

The 2 most widely used long-acting α-adrenoceptor blockers are phenoxybenzamine and doxazosine. Phenoxybenzamine is a noncompetitive α_1- and α_2-adrenoceptor blocker whereas doxazosine is a competitive selective α_1-adrenoceptor blocker. Phenoxybenzamine is usually started at a dose of 10 mg twice daily, followed by dose increments of 20 mg per day to a final dose of 1 mg/kg per day. Doxazosin is started at 2 mg per day with increasing the dose to 16 mg or even 32 mg per day. Dose titration is guided by symptoms, supine and standing blood pressure measurements, and side effects. Most prominent side effects of phenoxybenzamine include nasal congestion, orthostatic hypotension, and tachycardia. Doxazosine has less side effects, in particular less tachycardia. A concern of phenoxybenzamine is its propensity for prolonged postsurgical hypotension as compared with doxazosine, this being due to its long-lasting noncompetitive α-adrenoceptor blockade.

Because phenoxybenzamine crosses the placenta, it exposes the newborn to the risk of hypotension and respiratory depression.[52] Therefore monitoring the newborn for the first 3 postnatal days is recommended.[53] Doxazosine is also able to cross the placenta but no adverse events have been reported so far in newborns of mothers who were treated with this α-adrenoceptor blocker.[54] Both α-adrenoceptor blockers can be transferred to a small extent into maternal milk but there are no reports published that have shown adverse effects of breastfeeding in the newborns.[53] Balancing the efficacy and potential side effects of both α-adrenoceptor blockers in this special population, it is reasonable to use doxazosine as the preferred α-adrenoceptor blocker in pregnant patients with a PPGL.

A second kind of blockade in selected patients with a PPGL is β-adrenoceptor blockade with the aim to treat or to prevent tachyarrhythmias. To circumvent unopposed α-adrenoceptor–mediated vasoconstriction, a β-adrenoceptor blocking drug should only be started after some days of appropriate α-adrenergic blockade. Most commonly used drugs for this purpose are propranolol (40 mg 3 times daily) and atenolol (25–50 mg once daily).[4]

Several other drugs have been used in presurgical preparation, including calcium channel blockers and labetalol. There are insufficient data to support their safe use as monotherapy in pregnant patients with a PPGL. Labetalol for oral use has more potent β-adrenoceptor than α-adrenoceptor blocking efficacy, has been associated with reports of hypertensive crises and is not recommended. The catecholamine-synthesis inhibitor α-methylparatyrosine (metyrosine) is used at some centers as an adjunct to phenoxybenzamine, but this drug is contraindicated in pregnant patients.

An important consideration for presurgical preparation is the target blood pressure level. The recommended target blood pressure level of less than 130/80 mm Hg while seated and higher than 90 mm Hg systolic while standing for nonpregnant patients, may be too strict in pregnant women.[4] Strong vasodilation associated with large blood pressure reductions can jeopardize the uteroplacental circulation. There are however no reliable data that justify a strong recommendation concerning a specific blood pressure target in these patients. Despite the need to attain adequate α-adrenoceptor blockade in these patients, it may be prudent to target a blood pressure level of 140/90 mm Hg because that is also the recommended target for antihypertensive treatment in pregnancy by the European guideline for treatment of hypertension.[55]

As an adjunct to medication, increasing the intake of salt and fluid during presurgical preparation is essential to minimize the risk of postoperative hypotension.[4] Patients with a PPGL tend to have orthostatic hypotension which may even be enhanced by α-adrenoceptor blockade. Because hypertensive pregnant patients have a higher risk of (pre)eclampsia, it can be argued to manage these patients on an in-patient basis for close and optimal monitoring of blood pressure and volume status.

Similarly as in nonpregnant patients, a PPGL can present as a life-threatening emergency such as a hypertensive crisis, hypertensive encephalopathy, or cardiac ischemia.[8] It is important to keep in mind that such PPGL crisis may be invoked by different kinds of frequently used drugs, in particular peripartum. These include metoclopramide, steroids, and sympathomimetics.[56]

In pregnant patients the choice of drugs for therapeutic use in these acute settings is limited. The most widely available drugs for intravenous administration are rapid- and short-acting calcium channel blockers such as nicardipine and the vasodilator magnesium sulphate.[57] The latter is well known by anesthesiologists involved in obstetrics for treatment of eclampsia. This drug not only induces vasodilation but it is also supposed to inhibit catecholamine release and to reduce the sensitivity of α-adrenoceptors to catecholamines. Plasma magnesium levels should be monitored during continuous infusion. There is no evidence from any trial to support the use of any specific drug. Finally, in case of tachyarrhythmias a short-acting β-adrenoceptor blocker such as esmolol is available for intravenous use.

WHAT IS THE PREFERRED MODE OF DELIVERY IN A PATIENT HARBORING PHEOCHROMOCYTOMA OR PARAGANGLIOMA?

The ongoing debate about the optimal mode of delivery in patients with an active PPGL is fueled by the lack of reliable data to support either cesarean delivery or vaginal delivery. The available results from small series and case reports are critically dependent on whether the patient was properly pretreated or not. Warnings for the detrimental effects of labor during vaginal delivery, shifted clinical practice for a long time to cesarean delivery, a more controlled mode of delivery. One of the oldest studies showed that maternal mortality was lower (19%) than that of vaginal delivery (31%).[16] It is however unclear from this study whether the diagnosis of PPGL was made antenatally and whether all patients were properly pretreated. There are an increasing number of case reports showing an uneventful outcome also for vaginal delivery while on adrenergic blockade, sometimes even covered by spinal or epidural anesthesia.[19,58] The ultimate decision in elective cases about which mode of delivery to choose depends on several factors, such as parity, previous cesarean delivery, success of pretreatment, and the personal preference of the patient.[58] In most cases, cesarean delivery remains the preferred way of safe delivery. Epidural, general, or combined anesthetic techniques have been used successfully for cesarean delivery.[59]

In summary, the outcome of pregnancy in patients with a PPGL has considerably improved over the last decades. Obviously, more refined surgical and anesthesiologic techniques have contributed pivotally to this progress. In addition, the increase in proportion of patients in whom the diagnosis is made antenatally and thus treated in a timely manner has made a crucial contribution. However, this proportion seems to plateau now on about 70% to 75% of all patients, indicating that the diagnosis is still missed antenatally 1 out of every 3 to 4 patients. Because the antenatal diagnosis followed by proper treatment provides the best chance for successful outcome of pregnancy for mother and child, early awareness and recognition of the potential presence of a PPGL in a pregnant patient with hypertension is key for preventing premature loss of life. Once the diagnosis of a PPGL is confirmed, this specific group of patients should be managed by an experienced and dedicated multidisciplinary team.

REFERENCES

1. Lenders JW, Eisenhofer G, Mannelli M, et al. Phaeochromocytoma. Lancet 2005; 366(9486):665–75.

2. Mansmann G, Lau J, Balk E, et al. The clinically inapparent adrenal mass: update in diagnosis and management. Endocr Rev 2004;25(2):309–40.

3. Cawood TJ, Hunt PJ, O'Shea D, et al. Recommended evaluation of adrenal incidentalomas is costly, has high false-positive rates and confers a risk of fatal

cancer that is similar to the risk of the adrenal lesion becoming malignant; time for a rethink? Eur J Endocrinol 2009;161(4):513–27.

4. Lenders JW, Duh QY, Eisenhofer G, et al. Pheochromocytoma and paraganglioma: an endocrine society clinical practice guideline. J Clin Endocrinol Metab 2014;99(6):1915–42.

5. Lenders JW, Eisenhofer G. Pathophysiology and diagnosis of disorders of the adrenal medulla: focus on pheochromocytoma. Compr Physiol 2014;4(2):691–713.

6. Stolk RF, Bakx C, Mulder J, et al. Is the excess cardiovascular morbidity in pheochromocytoma related to blood pressure or to catecholamines? J Clin Endocrinol Metab 2013;98(3):1100–6.

7. Prejbisz A, Lenders JW, Eisenhofer G, et al. Mortality associated with phaeochromocytoma. Horm Metab Res 2013;45(2):154–8.

8. Riester A, Weismann D, Quinkler M, et al. Life-threatening events in patients with pheochromocytoma. Eur J Endocrinol 2015;173(6):757–64.

9. Favier J, Amar L, Gimenez-Roqueplo AP. Paraganglioma and phaeochromocytoma: from genetics to personalized medicine. Nat Rev Endocrinol 2015;11(2): 101–11.

10. Harper MA, Murnaghan GA, Kennedy L, et al. Phaeochromocytoma in pregnancy. Five cases and a review of the literature. Br J Obstet Gynaecol 1989; 96(5):594–606.

11. Harrington JL, Farley DR, van Heerden JA, et al. Adrenal tumors and pregnancy. World J Surg 1999;23(2):182–6.

12. Antonelli NM, Dotters DJ, Katz VL, et al. Cancer in pregnancy: a review of the literature. Part I. Obstet Gynecol Surv 1996;51(2):125–34.

13. Lenders JW. Pheochromocytoma and pregnancy: a deceptive connection. Eur J Endocrinol 2012;166(2):143–50.

14. Ahlawat SK, Jain S, Kumari S, et al. Pheochromocytoma associated with pregnancy: case report and review of the literature. Obstet Gynecol Surv 1999; 54(11):728–37.

15. Schenker JG, Chowers I. Pheochromocytoma and pregnancy. Review of 89 cases. Obstet Gynecol Surv 1971;26(11):739–47.

16. Schenker JG, Granat M. Phaeochromocytoma and pregnancy–an updated appraisal. Aust N Z J Obstet Gynaecol 1982;22(1):1–10.

17. Oishi S, Sato T. Pheochromocytoma in pregnancy: a review of the Japanese literature. Endocr J 1994;41(3):219–25.

18. Biggar MA, Lennard TW. Systematic review of phaeochromocytoma in pregnancy. Br J Surg 2013;100(2):182–90.

19. Wing LA, Conaglen JV, Meyer-Rochow GY, et al. Paraganglioma in pregnancy: a case series and review of the literature. J Clin Endocrinol Metab 2015;100(8): 3202–9.

20. Natrajan PG, McGarrigle HH, Lawrence DM, et al. Plasma noradrenaline and adrenaline levels in normal pregnancy and in pregnancy-induced hypertension. Br J Obstet Gynaecol 1982;89(12):1041–5.

21. O'Shaughnessy RW, Scott GD, Iams JD, et al. Plasma catecholamines in normal pregnancy and in pregnancies complicated by mild chronic hypertension. Clin Exp Hypertens B 1983;2(1):113–21.

22. Barron WM, Mujais SK, Zinaman M, et al. Plasma catecholamine responses to physiologic stimuli in normal human pregnancy. Am J Obstet Gynecol 1986; 154(1):80–4.

23. Oian P, Kjeldsen SE, Eide I, et al. Increased arterial catecholamines in preeclampsia. Acta Obstet Gynecol Scand 1986;65(6):613–7.

24. Khatun S, Kanayama N, Hossain B, et al. Increased concentrations of plasma epinephrine and norepinephrine in patients with eclampsia. Eur J Obstet Gynecol Reprod Biol 1996;69(2):61–7.
25. Saarikoski S. Fate of noradrenaline in the human foetoplacental unit. Acta Physiol Scand Suppl 1974;421:1–82.
26. Dahia PL, Hayashida CY, Strunz C, et al. Low cord blood levels of catecholamine from a newborn of a pheochromocytoma patient. Eur J Endocrinol 1994;130(3): 217–9.
27. Nguyen TT, Tseng YT, McGonnigal B, et al. Placental biogenic amine transporters: in vivo function, regulation and pathobiological significance. Placenta 1999;20(1):3–11.
28. Bzoskie L, Blount L, Kashiwai K, et al. Placental norepinephrine clearance: in vivo measurement and physiological role. Am J Physiol 1995;269(1 Pt 1):E145–9.
29. Slotkin TA, Seidler FJ. Adrenomedullary catecholamine release in the fetus and newborn: secretory mechanisms and their role in stress and survival. J Dev Physiol 1988;10(1):1–16.
30. Bramham K, Parnell B, Nelson-Piercy C, et al. Chronic hypertension and pregnancy outcomes: systematic review and meta-analysis. BMJ 2014;348:g2301.
31. Combs CA, Easterling TR, Schmucker BC, et al. Hemodynamic observations during paroxysmal hypertension in a pregnancy with pheochromocytoma. Obstet Gynecol 1989;74(3 Pt 2):439–41.
32. Neumann HP, Bausch B, McWhinney SR, et al. Germ-line mutations in nonsyndromic pheochromocytoma. N Engl J Med 2002;346(19):1459–66.
33. Oliva R, Angelos P, Kaplan E, et al. Pheochromocytoma in pregnancy: a case series and review. Hypertension 2010;55(3):600–6.
34. Prejbisz A, Lenders JW, Eisenhofer G, et al. Cardiovascular manifestations of phaeochromocytoma. J Hypertens 2011;29(11):2049–60.
35. Mannelli M, Bemporad D. Diagnosis and management of pheochromocytoma during pregnancy. J Endocrinol Invest 2002;25(6):567–71.
36. Seely EW, Ecker J. Chronic hypertension in pregnancy. Circulation 2014;129(11): 1254–61.
37. Eisenhofer G, Peitzsch M. Laboratory evaluation of pheochromocytoma and paraganglioma. Clin Chem 2014;60(12):1486–99.
38. Eisenhofer G, Prejbisz A, Peitzsch M, et al. Biochemical diagnosis of chromaffin cell tumors in patients at high and low risk of disease: plasma versus urinary free or deconjugated O-methylated catecholamine metabolites. Clin Chem 2018; 64(11):1646–56.
39. Eisenhofer G, Keiser H, Friberg P, et al. Plasma metanephrines are markers of pheochromocytoma produced by catechol-O-methyltransferase within tumors. J Clin Endocrinol Metab 1998;83(6):2175–85.
40. Yu R, Wei M. False positive test results for pheochromocytoma from 2000 to 2008. Exp Clin Endocrinol Diabetes 2010;118(9):577–85.
41. Lenders JW, Willemsen JJ, Eisenhofer G, et al. Is supine rest necessary before blood sampling for plasma metanephrines? Clin Chem 2007;53(2):352–4.
42. Darr R, Kuhn M, Bode C, et al. Accuracy of recommended sampling and assay methods for the determination of plasma-free and urinary fractionated metanephrines in the diagnosis of pheochromocytoma and paraganglioma: a systematic review. Endocrine 2017;56(3):495–503.
43. Eisenhofer G, Goldstein DS, Walther MM, et al. Biochemical diagnosis of pheochromocytoma: how to distinguish true- from false-positive test results. J Clin Endocrinol Metab 2003;88(6):2656–66.

44. Sarathi V, Lila AR, Bandgar TR, et al. Pheochromocytoma and pregnancy: a rare but dangerous combination. Endocr Pract 2010;16(2):300–9.
45. Ray JG, Vermeulen MJ, Bharatha A, et al. Association between MRI exposure during pregnancy and fetal and childhood outcomes. JAMA 2016;316(9):952–61.
46. Patenaude Y, Pugash D, Lim K, et al. The use of magnetic resonance imaging in the obstetric patient. J Obstet Gynaecol Can 2014;36(4):349–63.
47. Vanderveen KA, Thompson SM, Callstrom MR, et al. Biopsy of pheochromocytomas and paragangliomas: potential for disaster. Surgery 2009;146(6):1158–66.
48. Pearl J, Price R, Richardson W, et al. Guidelines for diagnosis, treatment, and use of laparoscopy for surgical problems during pregnancy. Surg Endosc 2011; 25(11):3479–92.
49. Fernandez-Cruz L, Taura P, Saenz A, et al. Laparoscopic approach to pheochromocytoma: hemodynamic changes and catecholamine secretion. World J Surg 1996;20(7):762–8 [discussion: 768].
50. Plouin PF, Amar L, Dekkers OM, et al. European Society of Endocrinology clinical practice guideline for long-term follow-up of patients operated on for a phaeochromocytoma or a paraganglioma. Eur J Endocrinol 2016;174(5):G1–10.
51. Burgess GE 3rd. Alpha blockade and surgical intervention of pheochromocytoma in pregnancy. Obstet Gynecol 1979;53(2):266–70.
52. Santeiro ML, Stromquist C, Wyble L. Phenoxybenzamine placental transfer during the third trimester. Ann Pharmacother 1996;30(11):1249–51.
53. Aplin SC, Yee KF, Cole MJ. Neonatal effects of long-term maternal phenoxybenzamine therapy. Anesthesiology 2004;100(6):1608–10.
54. Versmissen J, Koch BC, Roofthooft DW, et al. Doxazosin treatment of phaeochromocytoma during pregnancy: placental transfer and disposition in breast milk. Br J Clin Pharmacol 2016;82(2):568–9.
55. Williams B, Mancia G, Spiering W, et al. 2018 ESC/ESH guidelines for the management of arterial hypertension: the task force for the management of arterial hypertension of the European Society of Cardiology and the European Society of Hypertension: the task force for the management of arterial hypertension of the European Society of Cardiology and the European Society of Hypertension. J Hypertens 2018;36(10):1953–2041.
56. Eisenhofer G, Rivers G, Rosas AL, et al. Adverse drug reactions in patients with phaeochromocytoma: incidence, prevention and management. Drug Saf 2007; 30(11):1031–62.
57. James MF, Cronje L. Pheochromocytoma crisis: the use of magnesium sulfate. Anesth Analg 2004;99(3):680–6, table of contents.
58. van der Weerd K, van Noord C, Loeve M, et al. ENDOCRINOLOGY IN PREGNANCY: pheochromocytoma in pregnancy: case series and review of literature. Eur J Endocrinol 2017;177(2):R49–58.
59. Cammarano WB, Gray AT, Rosen MA, et al. Anesthesia for combined cesarean section and extra-adrenal pheochromocytoma resection: a case report and literature review. Int J Obstet Anesth 1997;6(2):112–7.

Pregnancy in Congenital Adrenal Hyperplasia

Nicole Reisch, MD

KEYWORDS

• Fertility • Pregnancy • Congenital adrenal hyperplasia • 21-Hydroxylase deficiency

KEY POINTS

- Fertility rates but not pregnancy rates in 21-hydroxylase deficiency (21-OHD) are reduced.
- Only use hydrocortisone or prednisolone for hormone replacement during pregnancy to avoid an effect on the fetus.
- Low-dose preconceptional glucocorticoids (hydrocortisone or prednisolone) and glucocorticoids administered during pregnancy normalize otherwise increased miscarriage rate in nonclassic 21-OHD.
- Knowledge of disease control parameters during pregnancy for monitoring purposes is lacking and needs further studies.
- Fludrocortisone may need to be added or the doses increased to enable conception in simple virilizing 21-OHD.
- Glucocorticoid dose may need to be increased 20% to 40% during the third trimester.
- Course and outcome of pregnancies are mostly uneventful.
- Stress-dose glucocorticoid treatment during delivery is required.

INTRODUCTION

Congenital adrenal hyperplasia (CAH) is a rare genetic cause of primary adrenal insufficiency.[1,2] It is a group of inborn errors of steroidogenesis affecting cortisol biosynthesis.[1] Decreased cortisol synthesis leads to increased adrenocorticotropic hormone (ACTH) concentrations and chronic adrenal stimulation causing hyperplasia. Levels of steroid precursors before the enzymatic block are grossly increased and show a characteristic pattern for each form of CAH. The most common form is 21-hydroxylase deficiency (21-OHD), accounting for more than 90% of all cases. According to newborn screening data, classic 21-OHD affects 1 in 10,000 to 1 in 15,000. It is associated with prenatally increased androgen levels causing various degrees of virilization of the external genitalia in girls, often requiring female reconstructive surgery.

Conflict of interest: The author has no conflict of interest.
Medizinische Klinik IV, Department of Endocrinology, Klinikum der Universität München, Ziemssenstraße 1, München 80336, Germany
E-mail address: nicole.reisch@med.uni-muenchen.de

Endocrinol Metab Clin N Am 48 (2019) 619–641
https://doi.org/10.1016/j.ecl.2019.05.011
0889-8529/19/© 2019 Elsevier Inc. All rights reserved.

The clinical phenotype includes the very severe salt wasting (SW) form with only 0% to 1% residual enzyme activity, the simple virilizing (SV) form with about 2% to 20% residual enzyme activity, and the mild nonclassic form.[3] Children with both the SW and SV forms are born with virilized external genitalia in girls, and this is known as the classic form. In addition to cortisol deficiency, the patients with the SW form also have aldosterone deficiency. Untreated neonates present with SW crises and die within the first weeks of life. Typically the nonclassic patients are not cortisol deficient but have slightly increased adrenal androgen levels leading to a polycystic ovary syndrome (PCOS)–like phenotype in girls with irregular cycles and subfertility, acne, and hirsutism.[4] Adrenal 11β-hydroxylase deficiency and type II 3β-hydroxysteroid dehydrogenase deficiency are other rare causes of virilizing CAH.[5]

Other very rare forms of CAH have a different phenotype with disrupted adrenal sexual steroid production caused by enzymatic or protein deficiencies, such as StAR (steroidogenic acute regulatory) deficiency, P450scc deficiency, and 17α-hydroxylase/17-20 lyase deficiency.[6] In these forms, patients show incomplete pubertal development and infertility in both sexes, whereas cortisol replacement therapy in the virilizing forms may lead to correction of adrenal hormone profile and enable spontaneous puberty and ideally fertility. Steroid P450 oxidoreductase deficiency (a flavoprotein donating electrons to P450 enzymes) can present with prenatal virilization of the external genitalia in girls because of a prenatal alternative pathway to androgens.[6] Shortly after birth this pathway closes and results in decreased sex steroid production and incomplete pubertal development.

This article focuses on female fertility and pregnancy in CAH caused by 21-OHD. It also briefly summarizes the available case reports on fertility and pregnancy in the very rare forms of CAH.

CLASSIC 21-HYDROXYLASE DEFICIENCY
Fecundity, Fertility, and Outcome of Pregnancies

On optimized glucocorticoid and mineralocorticoid replacement therapy, patients with classic 21-OHD experience normal spontaneous puberty and fecundity.[2] It could be shown that an equal pregnancy rate in classic 21-OHD can be achieved compared with the general population.[7] There was also no difference between the SW and the SV form of 21-OHD, with a pregnancy rate of 89% and 93% versus 95% in the general UK population.[7] This study clearly shows that those who wish to conceive do conceive. In contrast, studies clearly show that fertility rates are low because far fewer women seek motherhood in classic 21-OHD, particular in the SW form (only 11%).

In 1987, Mulaikal and colleagues[8] found substantially decreased fertility rates in classic CAH. Only half of the patients were heterosexually active, in 15 of 25 sexually active patients with the SV form 25 pregnancies resulted in 20 healthy children, whereas only 1 of 15 women with the SW from became pregnant. In this historical cohort, poor disease control seemed to be prevalent, with hirsutism and poor endocrine follow-up in 25% of patients. Furthermore, the vaginal introitus was reported to be inadequate for intercourse by 35% of patients. Premadwardhana and colleagues[9] described 8 pregnancies in 5 women (2 SV, 3 SW) out of a cohort of 16 women. At the time of publication, only 2 pregnancies resulted in live births, 5 were therapeutic abortions, and 1 was still awaiting delivery. The 2 live-born children were described as normal in their outcome. Lo and Grumbach[10] reported 7 pregnancies in 5 women with classic 21-OHD, 3 of them having the SW form. These pregnancies resulted in 4 live births, 1 spontaneous abortion, and 2 therapeutic abortions. A Finnish cohort of 29 patients with classic 21-OHD included 13 pregnancies in 9 women (1 SW, 8SV).[11] The total cohort consisted of 29 women, with 9 SW and 20 SV. Seven pregnancies were conceived naturally, 6 after human chorionic gonadotropin (hCG) stimulation. Krone and colleagues[12] reported 31 pregnancies in 18 women in a cohort of 122 women with 21-OHD (in 1 woman of 48 with the SW form, in 12 women of 64 with the SV form, and in 5 of 10 with the nonclassic form). The UK cohort published by Casteras and colleagues[7] investigated 34 pregnancies in 21 women out of a total cohort of 106 women with classic 21-OHD. The exact prevalence of pregnancies in CAH is unknown because available data are derived from small and mostly young cohorts, and there are no population-based data available on pregnancies and their outcomes. Because most adult patient cohorts are still young, with a median age of about 30 years, most patients are still in the reproductive phase and further pregnancies in this patient cohort have yet to happen.

However, the available studies on pregnancy outcome in CAH usually show uneventful courses of the pregnancies and good maternal and fetal outcomes. **Table 1** gives an overview of studies on pregnancies in classic 21-OHD.

FACTORS CONTRIBUTING TO LOWER FERTILITY

There are multiple factors contributing to reduced fertility in patients with 21-OHD. Hormonal factors play an essential role in conception as well as maintenance of pregnancy. In patients with poorly controlled disease there are two main agents interfering with the patients' reproductive potential: adrenal androgens and progesterone. Excess adrenal androgens are thought to directly suppress follicular development and compromise ovulation.[13] They cause endometrial molecular alterations and disrupt embryo implantation.[14] High levels of adrenal androgens also lead to increased gonadotropin-releasing hormone (GnRH) pulse frequency with increased luteinizing hormone (LH) concentrations relative to follicle-stimulating hormone (FSH).[15,16] As in PCOS, this results in increased androgen secretion by ovarian theca cells and cystic morphology of the ovaries. Progesterone oversecretion, as observed in poorly controlled patients, critically also interferes with female cycles.[17] Progesterone is known to be a key regulator of GnRH pulse frequency. Increased progesterone concentrations in patients with poorly controlled 21-OHD have been shown to be associated with reduced LH pulse frequency and amplitude, whereas LH pulse frequency was normal in well-controlled patients.[17] Increased progesterone concentrations have also been shown to be associated with oligoamenorrhea and infertility[18]; result in unfavorable cervical mucus; and disrupt endometrial thickening, ovulation, embryo implantation, and sperm migration. Increased progesterone concentration may also be observed in patients with otherwise optimal glucocorticoid replacement therapy.[7] In order to achieve pregnancy, slight glucocorticoid overtreatment therefore sometimes becomes necessary for a certain period of time.

Other reasons may be of a structural nature related to genital reconstructive surgery. Dissatisfaction with sexual life related to surgical complications may also contribute to low fertility.[19] The general consensus now is that 46,XX patients with 21-OHD are assigned female sex. In the past, clitoroplasty was regularly performed in early childhood, often together with vaginoplasty.[1] In adolescents, a second surgical intervention often corrected vaginal stenosis. Initial studies showed inadequate vaginal opening, impeding sexual intercourse in up to 50% of patients and potentially contributing to lower sexual activity in this patient cohort.[1] Clitoral surgery resulted in loss of sensitivity in many patients, contributing to sexual dissatisfaction.[19] It therefore has been questioned and indications have become more restrictive. Also, surgical methods have changed in the last decades.[1] Newer techniques preserving the clitoris

Table 1
Published case reports and case series of pregnancies in classic 21-hydroxylase deficiency with more than 3 pregnancies reported

Publication	Patients	Number of Pregnant Women and CAH Form	Total Number of Pregnancies	Number of Live Births	Abortions/Miscarriages	Mode of Conception/Induction of Pregnancy	Mode of Delivery	Maternal Outcome/Course of Pregnancy	Fetal Outcome
Klingensmith et al,[86] 1977	98	8 NR, 2 SW	15	9	3 SAB, 2 TAB, 1 died in childhood	NR	1 V, 9 C	NR	8 normal children, 1 born after 7 mo gestation and has mild spastic diplegia
Grant et al,[87] 1983	4	1 SV, 3 SW	1, 5	1, 4	0 but died in childhood, 1 TAB, 4 died in childhood	NR	1 C, 4 V	NR	1 lethal, 4 lethal
Mulaikal et al,[8] 1987	80	15 SV, 1 SW	25, 1	20	3 SAB, 2 TAB, 1 TAB	NR	4 V, >9 C	NR	Normal children
Kuhnle et al,[88] 1995	6	4 SV, 2 SW	4, 2	4, 2	0, but all 6 died in childhood	NR	NR	NR	6 lethal
Premawardhana et al,[9] 1997	16	2 SV, 3 SW	8	2	5 TAB	NR	1 V, 1 C, 1 awaiting delivery at publication	NR	Normal children

Study	N	Subtype			Outcome	Conception	Delivery	Maternal complications	Child outcomes
Lo et al,[89] 1999	4	1 SV 3 SW	2 5	1 3	1 SAB 2 TAB	Spontaneous IVF, 2 spontaneous	1 V 3 C	1 preeclampsia	3 normal children, 1 with fetal bradycardia and need for temporary mechanical ventilation with recovery without sequelae
Jääskeläinen et al,[11] 2000	29	8 SV 1 SW	12 1	10	2 SAB 1 TAB	6 spontaneous, 3 hMG + IUI, 3 hMG + hCG + IUI	3 V, 7 C	2 hepatosteatosis	Normal children, at birth, 2 IUGR, 1 asphyctic
Krone et al,[12] 2001	122	12 SV 1 SW 5 nonclassic	23 1 7	23 1 7	0	NR	10 V, 13 C 1 C 6 V, 1 C	Complicated pyelonephritis in 1 SV, preterm delivery in GW 32	Normal children, 2 born premature in GW 32 and 35, child born at GW 32 microcephalic, 5 children SGA

(continued on next page)

Table 1 (*continued*)

Publication	Patients	Number of Pregnant Women and CAH Form	Total Number of Pregnancies	Number of Live Births	Abortions/ Miscarriages	Mode of Conception/ Induction of Pregnancy	Mode of Delivery	Maternal Outcome/ Course of Pregnancy	Fetal Outcome
Hoepffner et al,[26] 2004	7	4 SV 3 SW	9	8	1 SAB	NR	8 C	Uncomplicated pregnancy	4 normal girls 4 normal boys
Dumic et al,[90] 2005	3	2 SV 1 SW	4	4	0	NR	1 V, 3 C	1 preeclampsia	4 normal girls
Kulshreshtha et al,[91] 2008	7	7 NR	13	7	2 SAB 4 TAB	NR	7 V	NR	7 normal children
Hagenfeldt et al,[92] 2008	62	29 SW 27 SV 6 other	31	25	2 SAB 4 TAB	5 increase in the glucocorticosteroid dose or addition of fludrocortisone induced ovulation and pregnancy; 2 IVF	21 C 4 V	5 gestational diabetes	19 normal girls 6 normal boys
Casteras et al,[7] 2009	106	13 SV 8 SW	20 14	14 12	1 SAB, 1 TAB, 2 premature babies died, 1 pregnancy ongoing 1 TAB, 1 ongoing pregnancy	14 spontaneous, 1 ovum donation, 4 clomiphene, 1 hMG 8 spontaneous, of which 2 after adrenalectomy	3 V, 9 C, 2 UKN 3 V, 3 C, 2 UKN	NR	3 preeclampsia

Study										
Yu et al,[93] 2012	8	5 SV 3 nonclassic	5 3	5 3	0 0	NR	NR	NR	5 C 3 C	NR	8 normal children
Remde et al,[65] 2016	39 (18 SW, 11 SV, 10 NC)	3 SW, 5 SV	6 (1 set of twins)	2 6	1 SAB 1 SAB	NR	NR	NR	2 C 5 C	Uncomplicated pregnancy	8 children born to patients with CAH weighed significantly less and were smaller than expected (the latter was not significant)
Slowikowska-Hilczer et al,[32] 2017	221	NR	NR	33	NR	28 spontaneous, 1 ovum donation, 4 ART	NR	NR	NR	NR	
Dörr et al,[94] 2018	50	50 NR	NR	117	22 SAB	NR	NR	NR	NR	67 CAH SW	

Abbreviations: ART, assisted reproductive treatment; C, cesarean section; FSH, follicle stimulating hormone; GW, gestational week; hMG, human menopausal gonadotropin; IUI, intrauterine insemination; IVF, in vitro fertilization; NR, not reported; SAB, spontaneous abortion; TAB, therapeutic abortion; UKN, unknown; V, vaginal delivery.

dorsal nerve, the vessel, and central mucosa that supply the glans are applied and show satisfying morphologic and functional results with regard to clitoral sensitivity and orgasm in most patients.[20,21] Furthermore, optimized vaginal dilation techniques are practised.[22] Nordenström and colleagues[19] reported overall good satisfaction with sexual function in a cohort of 62 adult women compared with age-matched controls. Only the most severe null genotype group, patients with no residual enzyme activity, scored lower for sexual function compared with healthy controls. Complications in surgery have been found to be associated with disease severity and are most common in the null genotype. Genotype-phenotype correlation in the most severe forms of 21-OHD has been described as high with regard to genital outcome (Prader stage).[23,24] This correlation seems to translate into sexual functioning in adulthood,[19] whereas health status in adult patients with 21-OHD otherwise seems not to be correlated with genotype.[3] Several changes in indication, timing, and method have been introduced and also vary from center to center. However, outcome studies are scarce, usually have low sample sizes, and show conflicting results.[22] Because of multiple methodological techniques and surgical approaches, comparison between studies often is impossible. Because surgical functional outcome can only be evaluated with a delay of about 20 years, current surgical approaches can only be evaluated after a long delay into the future.

Psychosexual factors may also influence women's sexual lives.[25–30] Psychosocial adaptation and coping strategies may be crucial for partnership and sexuality.[31] Studies again show variable outcome, with no difference in psychological adjustment in women with 21-OHD compared with controls.

Another common reason for sexual inactivity, the lack of a partner, also has to be considered. The dsd-LIFE study found that women with classic 21-OHD have fewer (heterosexual) partnerships, although again there may be multiple reasons, including anatomic causes, psychosexual, and psychosocial.[28,29,32–34]

Girls with 21-OHD have been shown to present with typical masculine behavior. Girls show a boyish play behavior, and adolescents show more interest in traditionally male sports and higher affinity for technical topics, rough and tumble play, and aggression, which is also reflected in a higher percentage of women in technical or traditionally male professions.[33,35–37] It is generally accepted that prenatal androgen exposure causes a probably dose-related masculinization of the central nervous system.[38] A higher percentage of homosexuality and bisexuality correlating with disease severity has also been reported and a potential causal relationship with prenatal androgen exposure has been discussed.[28–30,33,34] Surgical outcome with adequacy of the introitus has also been debated as a potentially underlying cause for homosexuality.[8] However, Nordenström and colleagues[19] showed that genital appearance did not correlate with sexual orientation but with the genotype and reported satisfaction with sexual life. Furthermore, the perception of stenosis of the introitus was not correlated with sexual orientation in the Swedish publication. Genital appearance also correlated with sexual satisfaction. Interestingly, the women's perceptions of their own genital appearance was worse than the perceptions of the health professionals.[19,33] Psychosexual health seems to contribute substantially to sexual satisfaction and fertility, emphasizing adequate psychological care and support for these patients throughout the lifetime.

It has also been described that up one-third of women with 21-OHD lack sexual interest and sexual fantasies.[27,28]

Patient education seems to be equally important but neglected. The dsd-LIFE study, a European multicenter study investigating clinical care of patients with various forms of disorders of sex differentiation, including CAH, focusing on the patients' perception, showed that patients may have an inadequate understanding of their fertility potential.[32] Fertility issues in this study had been discussed with only about 60% of the patients, and only half of the patients rated the given information as satisfied, 30% were neutral, and 20% were not satisfied. Most patients (60%) were aware of their fertility potential to have own biological children, whereas almost 30% did not know and 10% judged themselves as infertile.

PLACENTAL ROLE ON MATERNAL HYPERANDROGENISM AND STEROID METABOLISM

The fetoplacental unit has the ability to actively synthesize and metabolize steroid hormones and thus it actively controls the steroid milieu of the fetus. In women with 21-OHD, the mother is treated with glucocorticoids, and sometimes mineralocorticoids, firstly in order to replace those hormones and secondly to control the mothers' adrenal androgen excess. Hydrocortisone and prednisolone/prednisone are both inactivated by placental 11-β hydroxysteroid dehydrogenase type 2 (11β-HSD2) and thereby the fetus is protected from potentially supraphysiologic glucocorticoid doses taken by the mother.[39]

In contrast, dexamethasone crosses the placenta. It escapes the inactivation by placental 11β-HSD2 and thus suppresses the fetal adrenal cortex. Dexamethasone therefore should not be administered during pregnancy unless the effect on the fetus is desired within a prenatal treatment concept.

The fetus is able to produce cortisol as early as 50 days after conception.[40] Human fetal cortisol synthesis peaks as early as 8 to 10 weeks after conception. Placental progesterone can also be converted to cortisol; however, this activity has been noted later during gestation and probably accounts for less than 5% of circulating cortisol in the fetus, as shown in other primates.[41–43] Similarly, transplacental passage of maternal cortisol occurs, although also in substantially lower concentrations than those produced by the fetus during the first trimester. Total and free plasma cortisol, ACTH, corticotropin-releasing hormone (CRH), cortisol-binding globulin (CBG), and urinary-free cortisol levels increase during normal pregnancies.[44–47] The placenta can produce biologically active ACTH and CRH.[48] However, it is unclear whether placental CRH has clinically relevant effects on the pituitary-adrenal function in pregnancy. Following estrogen stimulation, CBG increases 3-fold to 4-fold and leads to higher total plasma cortisol concentrations and half-life of cortisol, and free cortisol level increases by the 11th week of gestation. Because there are no hypercortisolemic effects in healthy pregnancies and the circadian rhythm is maintained, the hypothalamic-pituitary-adrenal axis set point is altered and the tissue is more refractory to cortisol effects.

In healthy women androgen levels also increase during pregnancy.[49] However, the placenta protects the fetus from the mothers' potential androgen excess.[50] The placenta serves as a metabolic barrier in order not to expose the fetus to increased circulating maternal androgens and androgen precursors. Excess androgens from the mother are aromatized by the placenta to estradiol and estrone, thus effectively protecting the fetus from virilization effects. During the course of pregnancy, the aromatase concentration and activity in the human placenta increase substantially, up to 16.5-fold by term pregnancy.[51] The fetus therefore seems well protected from moderate maternal hyperandrogenism as in PCOS or pregnancy luteoma and poorly controlled CAH. There is 1 published case of a girl born with ambiguous external genitalia caused by maternal androgen excess in CAH in a mother with SV 21-OHD who ceased glucocorticoid replacement.[52] In other severe cases of maternal androgen excess, as seen in adrenal carcinoma or ovarian tumors, levels of maternal androgens and androgen precursors may also exceed placental aromatase activity, causing female fetal virilization.[53–56] Another factor conferring fetal protection from maternal gestational hyperandrogenism comes from estrogen-induced increased sex hormone–binding globulin concentrations, which reduce bioavailable testosterone although to a much lesser degree.[57] In pregnancy, increased progesterone level additionally exerts some antiandrogenic effects.[58] Furthermore, progesterone has antimineralocorticoid effects. The renin-angiotensin-aldosterone system increases after about the eighth week of gestation,[59,60] therefore higher doses of mineralocorticoid replacement may be necessary later in pregnancy.[61]

PRECONCEPTIONAL CONSIDERATIONS

Preconception endocrine counseling should mainly focus on 3 issues: first, optimized glucocorticoid and mineralocorticoid replacement, necessary in order to enable conception as well as maintenance of the pregnancy, should be discussed; second, the risk of having a child affected by 21-OHD and the possibility of experimental prenatal therapy; and third, glucocorticoid stress dosing during pregnancy in intercurrent illness, in case of hyperemesis and during labor and delivery.

To achieve normal ovulatory cycles and fertility, it seems important to suppress progesterone to less than 2 nmol/L.[7] Sometimes an 8-hourly application of prednisolone is helpful to achieve constantly suppressed progesterone concentrations,[7] and in our experience patients usually need to be slightly overtreated. Hoepffner and colleagues[26] showed that the addition of fludrocortisone even in cases of SV21-OHD and normal renin concentration may be beneficial. As for the pathophysiologic mechanism behind this, it is assumed that the progesterone excess may also originate from the aldosterone pathway.[7,26]

In rare cases in which adrenal androgens and progesterone cannot be sufficiently suppressed, bilateral adrenalectomy may restore cyclicity and successfully lead to pregnancy.[62–64] Bilateral adrenalectomy should be considered the ultima ratio because it abolishes any residual glucocorticoid and mineralocorticoid secretion, putting the patient at substantially higher risk for adrenal crises.[1] Before bilateral adrenalectomy, various methods of assisted reproductive techniques should be taken into account. Ovulation induction with clomiphene, gonadotropin therapy, or in vitro fertilization may be necessary for successful conception.[7] Once pregnancy is achieved, under continued glucocorticoid replacement therapy the course of pregnancy is usually uneventful,[12] although an increased rate (36%) of spontaneous miscarriages in all forms of 21-OHD has been described by Remde and colleagues[65] in 39 women. During pregnancy, close endocrine monitoring and cooperation between endocrinologist and obstetrician is recommended.

PRECONCEPTION GENETIC COUNSELING AND PRENATAL TREATMENT

Preconception genetic counseling should evaluate the risk of having a child affected with classic 21-OHD. Steroid 21-OHD follows an autosomal recessive trait with an incidence of 1 in 10,000 to 1 in 15,000,[66] which means that about 1 in 50 to 1 in 60 are carriers. In parents with carrier state and an index child, the risk of having another child with classic 21-OHD therefore is 25%. In mothers affected by classic 21-OHD and a partner who is a carrier for classic 21-OHD, the risk increases to 50%. Because of the good genotype-phenotype correlation, genotyping provides important information on expected disease severity. It therefore is recommended to genetically test the partner for carrier status of 21-OHD. In case of a risk of classic 21-OHD, prenatal therapy with dexamethasone has been shown to effectively ameliorate prenatal virilization in affected girls.[67] Dexamethasone is not inactivated by the placenta and thus should only be used if the effect on the fetus is wanted. However, this therapeutic option is under much debate, because potential long-term metabolic risks and adverse effects on cognition cannot be excluded. Dexamethasone not only suppresses the fetal adrenal gland but has potential adverse effects on brain development and metabolic programming. The literature describes teratogenic effects of high doses of dexamethasone administered to pregnant animals.[68,69] Prenatal glucocorticoid overexposure has been shown to result in postnatal hypertension; in programming effects on glucose and insulin homeostasis; in decreased glomerular filtration; and in the development of fatty liver in rats, sheep, and nonhuman primates.[68] In addition, multiple negative effects on brain development have been described: alteration of hippocampal structure in fetal rhesus macaques; reduced hippocampal growth and impairment of motor development in rodents; delayed maturation of neurons, myelination, glia, and vasculature in sheep; changes in adult behavior and affective function in rodents with impaired coping in aversive situations and depressionlike symptoms; and increased immobility and anxiety-related behavior.[68] Furthermore, 11β-HSD2 knockout mice have lower birth weight.[68] In pregnancies at risk for classic 21-OHD that have been treated prenatally with dexamethasone, there is also evidence for adverse effects of dexamethasone on cognition.[70]

Furthermore, prenatal therapy with dexamethasone is considered ethically highly problematic because it involves treatment of unaffected fetuses,[71–73] because, to be effective, treatment needs to be started very early in pregnancy (before gestational week 7) before diagnosis can be established. There is general agreement that, if parents opt for prenatal dexamethasone treatment, explicit patient information is needed about the nature of the treatment, and thus it should only be done with approval by ethical review boards and with the assurance of follow-up of treated cases because of uncertainty about the long-term impact of dexamethasone on the fetus/child.[1]

HORMONE REPLACEMENT THERAPY DURING PREGNANCY AND LACTATION

Hydrocortisone is the glucocorticoid of choice during pregnancy because it is efficiently metabolized by placental 11β-hydroxysteroid dehydrogenase type 2 and thus does not have an effect on the fetus.[39,44] In 21-OHD, regular cycles and ovulation can sometimes be established more effectively by prednisolone.[7] In such cases, prednisolone can be used during pregnancy as well because it also largely does not cross the placental barrier.

In general, the preconceptional glucocorticoid replacement dose with hydrocortisone or prednisolone remains unaltered during the first and most of the second trimester. Although the CBG increases in pregnancy, an increase of glucocorticoid replacement dose usually is not necessary at the beginning of pregnancy. In primary adrenal insufficiency, it is a common approach to increase the hydrocortisone dose by 20% to 40% in the third trimester, which usually translates into 5 to 7.5 mg of hydrocortisone.[74] In 21-OHD, the approach with regard to hormone replacement can be handled similarly. In adrenal insufficiency, glucocorticoid replacement therapy can only be monitored clinically.[75] The monitoring of clinical signs of overtreatment or undertreatment is just as important in 21-OHD. Overtreatment can lead to a higher risk of glucose intolerance of gestational diabetes, hypertension, excessive weight gain, bruising, edema, or even preeclampsia. In contrast, undertreatment may put the patient at risk for hyperemesis and adrenal crises. In 21-OHD, in most centers disease control is monitored mainly by androstenedione and 17-hydroxyprogesterone in serum because this is usually available.[76] In addition, these steroids may be monitored in saliva or the steroid metabolome may be monitored in urine. In pregnancy, pronounced adaptations in pregnancy-related hormone concentrations take place, characterized by increased levels of multiple circulating steroid hormones.[49] Levels of all the steroid hormones used for disease monitoring in 21-OHD increase dramatically during pregnancy. Therefore, the usual reference ranges to monitor hormonal control cannot be applied during pregnancy. Levels of steroid 17-hydroxyprgoesterone increase throughout pregnancy, whereas androstenedione increases up to 80% by gestation week 12 and remains at that level for the remainder of the pregnancy.[49] It is essential to apply trimester-specific reference intervals in order to interpret hormone concentrations during pregnancy.[49]

Progesterone level is increased throughout pregnancy, with concentrations about 4 times higher in the third trimester compared with the first trimester. Because progesterone has an anti-mineralocorticoid effect, higher doses of fludrocortisone may be required in the third trimester.[61] Hydrocortisone has a mineralocorticoid effect, with about 40 mg of hydrocortisone equaling 0.1 mg of fludrocortisone. Because the hydrocortisone is increased toward the end of pregnancy, the additional requirement for fludrocortisone is usually already covered and it only needs to be slightly increased in the third trimester. Fludrocortisone dose needs to be monitored on clinical grounds based on blood pressure as well as serum potassium concentrations. Because plasma renin level profoundly changes during pregnancy,[60] it cannot be used as a reliable disease-monitoring marker.

Follow-up visits once every trimester seem reasonable, with clinical checkup and the aim of keeping androstenedione and testosterone levels in trimester-specific reference ranges, although there is a lack of evidence for how best to monitor 21-OHD during pregnancy.

MANAGEMENT OF ADRENAL CRISES

Adrenal crises are also a problem in adult 21-OHD. There is no consensus on the definition of adrenal crisis.[77] Adrenal crisis generally describes a situation in which the increased demand for circulating cortisol cannot be met.

A few studies have investigated the prevalence of adrenal crises in 21-OHD and these found 5 to 7 adrenal crisis per 100 patient years, and that children are at a substantially higher risk of experiencing adrenal crises than adults.[78,79] There are no data on the specific prevalence of adrenal crises in 21-OHD during pregnancy. Hahner and colleagues[80] prospectively investigated 423 patients with adrenal insufficiency over 2 years with regard to the incidence and causes of adrenal crises. In 1 patient, pregnancy triggered an adrenal crisis. Another German study investigated 93 patients with adrenal insufficiency, including 39 with 21-OHD, describing 1 adrenal crisis during pregnancy in this cohort.[65] A potential trigger of adrenal crises specific for pregnancy is hyperemesis. Patient and partner education on sick-day rules are important measures to prevent adrenal crises. Although adrenal crises management in pregnancy does not differ from regular adrenal crises handling, it is advised to reevaluate and refresh the patient's knowledge of emergency recommendations in this situation. The patients may feel more insecure because of pregnancy and can be reassured about how to act and encouraged to apply the sick-day rules. In addition, the patient's emergency kit should be checked again.

STRESS DOSING DURING LABOR AND DELIVERY

Labor and delivery are major physical stress situations and require glucocorticoid dose adjustment.[81] Swedish data showed that serum cortisol concentrations are higher in women during vaginal delivery compared with elective caesarean section, indicating higher stress levels.[81] This finding indicates that stress dosing in elective caesarean sections might be reduced. More precise guidelines for stress dosing during labor and delivery need to be established. According to international guidelines, clinicians currently advise patients to take 50 mg of hydrocortisone orally when labor starts and repeat this every 6 hours. On arrival in the hospital, 200 mg of hydrocortisone should be given intravenously over 24 hours. In case of uneventful delivery, on the first postpartal day the authors recommend reduction of the hydrocortisone dosage to 100 mg/d, divided into 4 doses; for example, 30, 30, 20, and 20 mg of hydrocortisone. On the second day after giving birth, we reduce the hydrocortisone dose to 50 mg (20, 20, 10 mg), with further dose reduction in the next few days to 35 mg total per day. We advise prompt consultation in our outpatient clinic after delivery, with clinical evaluation and potential further dose adaptation.

Breastfeeding can be encouraged in women on cortisol replacement therapy. Although hydrocortisone and prednisolone are both excreted in breast milk, the amounts of glucocorticoids are extremely low, so the exposure of babies to glucocorticoids from breastmilk is negligible and therefore unlikely to be harmful.[82,83] Even when high doses of prednisolone in lactating women were found, only negligible concentrations were found in the breast milk. The authors advise mothers to breastfeed their babies and take the hydrocortisone doses, when possible, immediately after breastfeeding.

OUTCOME OF PREGNANCIES

The outcomes of most pregnancies in 21-OHD are good, with healthy children born (see **Table 1**). The rate of small-for-gestational-age children seems to be increased. However, psychomotor and somatic long-term development of the children seem to be within the range of the normal population and their families. Follow-up in the study by Krone and colleagues[12] was up to 5 years in 31 children, 5 to 10 years in 7 children, and 18 children were older than 10 years.

NONCLASSIC 21-HYDROXYLASE DEFICIENCY

Most women with nonclassic 21-OHD (NC-21-OHD) have been shown to conceive spontaneously despite adrenal and ovarian androgen excess.[84,85] Rates for spontaneous conception are 69% without glucocorticoid treatment and 86% with low-dose glucocorticoid treatment. In nonclassic CAH, 2 studies showed an increased rate of spontaneous miscarriage in untreated NC-21-OHD.[84,85] This increased rate of pregnancy loss has been shown to be normalized with glucocorticoid treatment. The rate of ectopic pregnancy, preterm birth, stillbirth, or twins and multiple pregnancies was equal in treated versus untreated women with NC-21-OHD. The main cause of infertility or subfertility in NC-21-OHD is anovulation, which can be overcome by ovulation induction. Another reason is that persistently increased progesterone concentrations (of adrenal origin), as in classic 21-OHD, make the cervical mucus thicker and lead to hypotrophic or atrophic endometrium. Based on these data, low-dose glucocorticoid treatment with hydrocortisone or prednisolone can be recommended in patients with NC-21-OHD.

OTHER FORMS OF CONGENITAL ADRENAL HYPERPLASIA

There are case reports of fertility or pregnancy outcome in rarer forms of CAH. These reports are summarized in **Table 2**.

Table 2
Published cases of pregnancy in rare forms of congenital adrenal hyperplasia (other than 21-hydroxylase deficiency)

Publication	Number of Patients	Number of Pregnant Women and CAH Form	Total Number of Pregnancies	Number of Live Births	Number of Abortions/ Miscarriages	Mode of Conception/ Induction of Pregnancy	Mode of Delivery	Maternal Outcome/ Course of Pregnancy	Fetal Outcome
CAH Caused by 11β-Hydroxylase Deficiency									
Hazard et al,[95] 1980	6	3 11β-hydroxylase deficiency	3	3	0	NR	NR	NR	NR
Simm & Zacharin,[96] 2007	1	1 11β-hydroxylase deficiency	1	1	0	Clomiphene	1 C	During the pregnancy increasing clinical and biochemical virilization	1 normal boy
CAH Caused by 17α-Hydroxylase Deficiency									
Rabinovici et al,[97] 1989	1	1 17α-hydroxylase deficiency	0	0	0 (no pregnancy achieved)	IVF, prednisone 5 10 mg, GnRHa 1.2–1.5 mg, FSH, hCG 10,000 IU × 2	0	NR	Arrest of 2 of the 3 embryos at cleavage stage
Pellicer et al,[98] 1991	1	1 17α-hydroxylase deficiency	0	0	0 (no pregnancy achieved)	IVF, FSH 300 IU, hCG 10,000 IU	0	NR	2 PN × 11; no implantation with fresh or frozen ET
Neuwinger et al,[99] 1996	1	1 17α-hydroxylase deficiency	0	0	0 (no pregnancy achieved)	IVF, vaginal T 200–400 mg, FSH 300–550 IU, hMG 150–225 IU, hCG 10,000 IU	0	NR	Six oocytes retrieved with no fertilization

Reference	n	Diagnosis				Treatment			Outcome
Levran et al,[100] 2003	4	1 (partial 17,20-desmolase and 17α-hydroxylase deficiency)	1	3	0	IVF, transfer of cryopreserved embryos, dexamethasone and GnRH agonists, hMGs, and hCG during her controlled ovarian hyperstimulation	NR	NR	NR; No implantation
Matsuzaki et al,[101] 2000	1	17α-hydroxylase deficiency/17,20-lyase deficiency	0	0	0 no pregnancy achieved	FSH 225 IU, hCG 10,000 IU	0	0	NR
Bianchi et al,[102] 2016	1	17α-hydroxylase deficiency	1	1	0	Transfer of 2 cryopreserved embryos	1 C	Preeclampsia, gestational diabetes, cholestasis gravidarum, cellulitis of the lower right extremity, emergency cesarean section was performed because of acute fetal distress, puerperium uneventful	1 normal boy
Kitajima et al,[103] 2018	1	17α-hydroxylase deficiency	2	2	0	IVF with controlled ovarian stimulation	NR	NR	NR
Congenital Lipoid Adrenal Hyperplasia (StAR Deficiency)									
Khoury et al,[104] 2009	1	Lipoid CAH	3	3	1 SAB	Clomiphene stimulation	2 V twins 1 V	Uncomplicated pregnancy	2 normal boys 1 normal girl
Sertedaki et al,[105] 2009	1	Lipoid CAH	1	1	0	Ovarian stimulation, oocyte retrieval followed by IVF, additional estrogen support until placental function initiation	1 C	Uneventful pregnancy	1 normal girl

(continued on next page)

Table 2
(continued)

Publication	Number of Patients	Number of Pregnant Women and CAH Form	Total Number of Pregnancies	Number of Live Births	Abortions/ Miscarriages	Mode of Conception/ Induction of Pregnancy	Mode of Delivery	Maternal Outcome/ Course of Pregnancy	Fetal Outcome
Albarel et al,[106] 2016	1	1 lipoid CAH	1	1	0	Clomiphene stimulation, IVF; transfer of cryopreserved embryos	NR	Uneventful pregnancy	1 normal girl
P450 Oxidoreductase Deficiency									
Song et al,[107] 2018	1	1 P450 oxidoreductase deficiency	1	1	0	IVF, frozen embryo was transferred during hormone replacement therapy	NR	NR	1 normal child

Abbreviations: FSH follicle-stimulating hormone; GnRHa, gonadotropin-releasing hormone agonist; T, testosterone.

ACKNOWLEDGMENTS

This work was supported by the Deutsche Forschungsgemeinschaft (Heisenberg Professorship 325768017 and within the CRC/Transregio 205/1 "The Adrenal: Central Relay in Health and Disease" to N. Reisch).

REFERENCES

1. Speiser PW, Arlt W, Auchus RJ, et al. Congenital adrenal hyperplasia due to steroid 21-hydroxylase deficiency: an endocrine society clinical practice guideline. J Clin Endocrinol Metab 2018;103(11):4043–88.
2. El-Maouche D, Arlt W, Merke DP. Congenital adrenal hyperplasia. Lancet 2017; 390(10108):2194–210.
3. Krone N, Rose IT, Willis DS, et al. Genotype-phenotype correlation in 153 adult patients with congenital adrenal hyperplasia due to 21-hydroxylase deficiency: analysis of the United Kingdom Congenital adrenal Hyperplasia Adult Study Executive (CaHASE) cohort. J Clin Endocrinol Metab 2013;98(2):E346–54.
4. Nordenstrom A, Falhammar H. Management of endocrine disease: Diagnosis and management of the patient with non-classic CAH due to 21-hydroxylase deficiency. Eur J Endocrinol 2018. [Epub ahead of print].
5. Krone N, Arlt W. Genetics of congenital adrenal hyperplasia. Best Pract Res Clin Endocrinol Metab 2009;23(2):181–92.
6. Miller WL, Auchus RJ. The molecular biology, biochemistry, and physiology of human steroidogenesis and its disorders. Endocr Rev 2011;32(1):81–151.
7. Casteras A, De Silva P, Rumsby G, et al. Reassessing fecundity in women with classical congenital adrenal hyperplasia (CAH): normal pregnancy rate but reduced fertility rate. Clin Endocrinol (Oxf) 2009;70(6):833–7.
8. Mulaikal RM, Migeon CJ, Rock JA. Fertility rates in female patients with congenital adrenal hyperplasia due to 21-hydroxylase deficiency. N Engl J Med 1987; 316(4):178–82.
9. Premawardhana LD, Hughes IA, Read GF, et al. Longer term outcome in females with congenital adrenal hyperplasia (CAH): the Cardiff experience. Clin Endocrinol (oxf) 1997;46(3):327–32.
10. Lo JC, Grumbach MM. Pregnancy outcomes in women with congenital virilizing adrenal hyperplasia. Endocrinol Metab Clin North Am 2001;30(1):207–29.
11. Jääskeläinen J, Hippelainen M, Kiekara O, et al. Child rate, pregnancy outcome and ovarian function in females with classical 21-hydroxylase deficiency. Acta Obstet Gynecol Scand 2000;79(8):687–92.
12. Krone N, Wachter I, Stefanidou M, et al. Mothers with congenital adrenal hyperplasia and their children: outcome of pregnancy, birth and childhood. Clin Endocrinol (Oxf) 2001;55(4):523–9.
13. Walters KA, Handelsman DJ. Role of androgens in the ovary. Mol Cell Endocrinol 2018;465:36–47.
14. Simitsidellis I, Saunders PTK, Gibson DA. Androgens and endometrium: New insights and new targets. Mol Cell Endocrinol 2018;465:48–60.
15. Hague WM, Adams J, Rodda C, et al. The prevalence of polycystic ovaries in patients with congenital adrenal hyperplasia and their close relatives. Clin Endocrinol (Oxf) 1990;33(4):501–10.
16. Burt Solorzano CM, McCartney CR, Blank SK, et al. Hyperandrogenaemia in adolescent girls: origins of abnormal gonadotropin-releasing hormone secretion. BJOG 2010;117(2):143–9.

17. Bachelot A, Chakhtoura Z, Plu-Bureau G, et al. Influence of hormonal control on LH pulsatility and secretion in women with classical congenital adrenal hyperplasia. Eur J Endocrinol 2012;167(4):499–505.

18. Holmes-Walker DJ, Conway GS, Honour JW, et al. Menstrual disturbance and hypersecretion of progesterone in women with congenital adrenal hyperplasia due to 21-hydroxylase deficiency. Clin Endocrinol (Oxf) 1995;43(3):291–6.

19. Nordenström A, Frisén L, Falhammar H, et al. Sexual function and surgical outcome in women with congenital adrenal hyperplasia due to CYP21A2 deficiency: clinical perspective and the patients' perception. J Clin Endocrinol Metab 2010;95(8):3633–40.

20. Sircili MH, de Mendonca BB, Denes FT, et al. Anatomical and functional outcomes of feminizing genitoplasty for ambiguous genitalia in patients with virilizing congenital adrenal hyperplasia. Clinics (Sao Paulo) 2006;61(3):209–14.

21. Gomes LG, Bachega T, Mendonca BB. Classic congenital adrenal hyperplasia and its impact on reproduction. Fertil Steril 2019;111(1):7–12.

22. Almasri J, Zaiem F, Rodriguez-Gutierrez R, et al. Genital reconstructive surgery in females with congenital adrenal hyperplasia: a systematic review and meta-analysis. J Clin Endocrinol Metab 2018;103(11):4089–96.

23. Krone N, Braun A, Roscher AA, et al. Predicting phenotype in steroid 21-hydroxylase deficiency? Comprehensive genotyping in 155 unrelated, well defined patients from southern Germany. J Clin Endocrinol Metab 2000;85(3):1059–65.

24. Jaaskelainen J, Levo A, Voutilainen R, et al. Population-wide evaluation of disease manifestation in relation to molecular genotype in steroid 21-hydroxylase (CYP21) deficiency: good correlation in a well defined population. J Clin Endocrinol Metab 1997;82(10):3293–7.

25. Reichman DE, White PC, New MI, et al. Fertility in patients with congenital adrenal hyperplasia. Fertil Steril 2014;101(2):301–9.

26. Hoepffner W, Schulze E, Bennek J, et al. Pregnancies in patients with congenital adrenal hyperplasia with complete or almost complete impairment of 21-hydroxylase activity. Fertil Steril 2004;81(5):1314–21.

27. Meyer-Bahlburg HF, Dolezal C, Baker SW, et al. Gender development in women with congenital adrenal hyperplasia as a function of disorder severity. Arch Sex Behav 2006;35(6):667–84.

28. Meyer-Bahlburg HF, Dolezal C, Baker SW, et al. Sexual orientation in women with classical or non-classical congenital adrenal hyperplasia as a function of degree of prenatal androgen excess. Arch Sex Behav 2008;37(1):85–99.

29. Zucker KJ, Bradley SJ, Oliver G, et al. Psychosexual development of women with congenital adrenal hyperplasia. Horm Behav 1996;30(4):300–18.

30. Hines M, Brook C, Conway GS. Androgen and psychosexual development: core gender identity, sexual orientation and recalled childhood gender role behavior in women and men with congenital adrenal hyperplasia (CAH). J Sex Res 2004;41(1):75–81.

31. Berenbaum SA, Korman Bryk K, Duck SC, et al. Psychological adjustment in children and adults with congenital adrenal hyperplasia. J Pediatr 2004;144(6):741–6.

32. Slowikowska-Hilczer J, Hirschberg AL, Claahsen-van der Grinten H, et al. Fertility outcome and information on fertility issues in individuals with different forms of disorders of sex development: findings from the dsd-LIFE study. Fertil Steril 2017;108(5):822–31.

33. Frisen L, Nordenström A, Falhammar H, et al. Gender role behavior, sexuality, and psychosocial adaptation in women with congenital adrenal hyperplasia due to CYP21A2 deficiency. J Clin Endocrinol Metab 2009;94(9):3432–9.

34. Dittmann RW, Kappes ME, Kappes MH. Sexual behavior in adolescent and adult females with congenital adrenal hyperplasia. Psychoneuroendocrinology 1992;17(2–3):153–70.

35. Nordenstrom A, Servin A, Bohlin G, et al. Sex-typed toy play behavior correlates with the degree of prenatal androgen exposure assessed by CYP21 genotype in girls with congenital adrenal hyperplasia. J Clin Endocrinol Metab 2002;87(11): 5119–24.

36. Pasterski VL, Geffner ME, Brain C, et al. Prenatal hormones and postnatal socialization by parents as determinants of male-typical toy play in girls with congenital adrenal hyperplasia. Child Dev 2005;76(1):264–78.

37. Berenbaum SA, Duck SC, Bryk K. Behavioral effects of prenatal versus postnatal androgen excess in children with 21-hydroxylase-deficient congenital adrenal hyperplasia. J Clin Endocrinol Metab 2000;85(2):727–33.

38. Auyeung B, Lombardo MV, Baron-Cohen S. Prenatal and postnatal hormone effects on the human brain and cognition. Pflugers Arch 2013;465(5):557–71.

39. Benediktsson R, Calder AA, Edwards CR, et al. Placental 11 beta-hydroxysteroid dehydrogenase: a key regulator of fetal glucocorticoid exposure. Clin Endocrinol (Oxf) 1997;46(2):161–6.

40. Goto M, Piper Hanley K, Marcos J, et al. In humans, early cortisol biosynthesis provides a mechanism to safeguard female sexual development. J Clin Invest 2006;116(4):953–60.

41. Macnaughton MC, Taylor T, McNally EM, et al. The effect of synthetic ACTH on the metabolism of [4-14C]-progesterone by the previable human fetus. J Steroid Biochem 1977;8(5):499–504.

42. Pepe GJ, Albrecht ED. The utilization of placental substrates for cortisol synthesis by the baboon fetus near term. Steroids 1980;35(5):591–7.

43. Ducsay CA, Stanczyk FZ, Novy MJ. Maternal and fetal production rates of progesterone in rhesus macaques: placental transfer and conversion to cortisol. Endocrinology 1985;117(3):1253–8.

44. Lindsay JR, Nieman LK. The hypothalamic-pituitary-adrenal axis in pregnancy: challenges in disease detection and treatment. Endocr Rev 2005;26(6):775–99.

45. Jung C, Ho JT, Torpy DJ, et al. A longitudinal study of plasma and urinary cortisol in pregnancy and postpartum. J Clin Endocrinol Metab 2011;96(5): 1533–40.

46. Mastorakos G, Ilias I. Maternal and fetal hypothalamic-pituitary-adrenal axes during pregnancy and postpartum. Ann N Y Acad Sci 2003;997:136–49.

47. Nolten WE, Lindheimer MD, Rueckert PA, et al. Diurnal patterns and regulation of cortisol secretion in pregnancy. J Clin Endocrinol Metab 1980;51(3):466–72.

48. Petraglia F, Sawchenko PE, Rivier J, et al. Evidence for local stimulation of ACTH secretion by corticotropin-releasing factor in human placenta. Nature 1987; 328(6132):717–9.

49. Soldin OP, Guo T, Weiderpass E, et al. Steroid hormone levels in pregnancy and 1 year postpartum using isotope dilution tandem mass spectrometry. Fertil Steril 2005;84(3):701–10.

50. Sanderson JT. Placental and fetal steroidogenesis. Methods Mol Biol 2009;550: 127–36.

51. Kitawaki J, Inoue S, Tamura T, et al. Increasing aromatase cytochrome P-450 level in human placenta during pregnancy: studied by immunohistochemistry and enzyme-linked immunosorbent assay. Endocrinology 1992;130(5):2751–7.

52. Kai H, Nose O, Iida Y, et al. Female pseudohermaphroditism caused by maternal congenital adrenal hyperplasia. J Pediatr 1979;95(3):418–20.

53. Morris LF, Park S, Daskivich T, et al. Virilization of a female infant by a maternal adrenocortical carcinoma. Endocr Pract 2011;17(2):e26–31.

54. Fuller PJ, Pettigrew IG, Pike JW, et al. An adrenal adenoma causing virilization of mother and infant. Clin Endocrinol (Oxf) 1983;18(2):143–53.

55. Masarie K, Katz V, Balderston K. Pregnancy luteomas: clinical presentations and management strategies. Obstet Gynecol Surv 2010;65(9):575–82.

56. Wadzinski TL, Altowaireb Y, Gupta R, et al. Luteoma of pregnancy associated with nearly complete virilization of genetically female twins. Endocr Pract 2014;20(2):e18–23.

57. Kerlan V, Nahoul K, Le Martelot MT, et al. Longitudinal study of maternal plasma bioavailable testosterone and androstanediol glucuronide levels during pregnancy. Clin Endocrinol (Oxf) 1994;40(2):263–7.

58. Mauvais-Jarvis P, Kuttenn F, Baudot N. Inhibition of testosterone conversion to dihydrotestosterone in men treated percutaneously by progesterone. J Clin Endocrinol Metab 1974;38(1):142–7.

59. West CA, Sasser JM, Baylis C. The enigma of continual plasma volume expansion in pregnancy: critical role of the renin-angiotensin-aldosterone system. Am J Physiol Ren Physiol 2016;311(6):F1125–34.

60. Wilson M, Morganti AA, Zervoudakis I, et al. Blood pressure, the renin-aldosterone system and sex steroids throughout normal pregnancy. Am J Med 1980;68(1):97–104.

61. Quinkler M, Meyer B, Oelkers W, et al. Renal inactivation, mineralocorticoid generation, and 11beta-hydroxysteroid dehydrogenase inhibition ameliorate the antimineralocorticoid effect of progesterone in vivo. J Clin Endocrinol Metab 2003;88(8):3767–72.

62. Ogilvie CM, Rumsby G, Kurzawinski T, et al. Outcome of bilateral adrenalectomy in congenital adrenal hyperplasia: one unit's experience. Eur J Endocrinol 2006; 154(3):405–8.

63. Van Wyk JJ, Ritzen EM. The role of bilateral adrenalectomy in the treatment of congenital adrenal hyperplasia. J Clin Endocrinol Metab 2003;88(7):2993–8.

64. MacKay D, Nordenstrom A, Falhammar H. Bilateral adrenalectomy in congenital adrenal hyperplasia: a systematic review and meta-analysis. J Clin Endocrinol Metab 2018. [Epub ahead of print].

65. Remde H, Zopf K, Schwander J, et al. Fertility and pregnancy in primary adrenal insufficiency in Germany. Horm Metab Res 2016;48(5):306–11.

66. Hannah-Shmouni F, Chen W, Merke DP. Genetics of congenital adrenal hyperplasia. Endocrinol Metab Clin North Am 2017;46(2):435–58.

67. New MI, Carlson A, Obeid J, et al. Prenatal diagnosis for congenital adrenal hyperplasia in 532 pregnancies. J Clin Endocrinol Metab 2001;86(12):5651–7.

68. Khulan B, Drake AJ. Glucocorticoids as mediators of developmental programming effects. Best Pract Res Clin Endocrinol Metab 2012;26(5):689–700.

69. Witchel SF, Miller WL. Prenatal treatment of congenital adrenal hyperplasia-not standard of care. J Genet Couns 2012;21(5):615–24.

70. Miller WL. Fetal endocrine therapy for congenital adrenal hyperplasia should not be done. Best Pract Res Clin Endocrinol Metab 2015;29(3):469–83.

71. Miller WL, Witchel SF. Prenatal treatment of congenital adrenal hyperplasia: risks outweigh benefits. Am J Obstet Gynecol 2013;208(5):354–9.
72. Karlsson L, Nordenstrom A, Hirvikoski T, et al. Prenatal dexamethasone treatment in the context of at risk CAH pregnancies: long-term behavioral and cognitive outcome. Psychoneuroendocrinology 2018;91:68–74.
73. Hirvikoski T, Nordenstrom A, Wedell A, et al. Prenatal dexamethasone treatment of children at risk for congenital adrenal hyperplasia: the Swedish experience and standpoint. J Clin Endocrinol Metab 2012;97(6):1881–3.
74. Lebbe M, Arlt W. What is the best diagnostic and therapeutic management strategy for an Addison patient during pregnancy? Clin Endocrinol (Oxf) 2013;78(4): 497–502.
75. Reisch N, Arlt W. Fine tuning for quality of life: 21st century approach to treatment of Addison's disease. Endocrinol Metab Clin North Am 2009;38(2):407–18, ix-x.
76. Reisch N. Substitution therapy in adult patients with congenital adrenal hyperplasia. Best Pract Res Clin Endocrinol Metab 2015;29(1):33–45.
77. Rushworth RL, Torpy DJ, Falhammar H. Adrenal crises: perspectives and research directions. Endocrine 2017;55(2):336–45.
78. Odenwald B, Nennstiel-Ratzel U, Dörr HG, et al. Children with classic congenital adrenal hyperplasia experience salt loss and hypoglycemia: evaluation of adrenal crises during the first 6 years of life. Eur J Endocrinol 2016;174(2):177–86.
79. Reisch N, Willige M, Kohn D, et al. Frequency and causes of adrenal crises over lifetime in patients with 21-hydroxylase deficiency. Eur J Endocrinol 2012; 167(1):35–42.
80. Hahner S, Spinnler C, Fassnacht M, et al. High incidence of adrenal crisis in educated patients with chronic adrenal insufficiency: a prospective study. J Clin Endocrinol Metab 2015;100(2):407–16.
81. Stjernholm YV, Nyberg A, Cardell M, et al. Circulating maternal cortisol levels during vaginal delivery and elective cesarean section. Arch Gynecol Obstet 2016;294(2):267–71.
82. McKenzie SA, Selley JA, Agnew JE. Secretion of prednisolone into breast milk. Arch Dis Child 1975;50(11):894–6.
83. Ost L, Wettrell G, Bjorkhem I, et al. Prednisolone excretion in human milk. J Pediatr 1985;106(6):1008–11.
84. Bidet M, Bellanné-Chantelot C, Galand-Portier MB, et al. Fertility in women with nonclassical congenital adrenal hyperplasia due to 21-hydroxylase deficiency. J Clin Endocrinol Metab 2010;95(3):1182–90.
85. Moran C, Azziz R, Weintrob N, et al. Reproductive outcome of women with 21-hydroxylase-deficient nonclassic adrenal hyperplasia. J Clin Endocrinol Metab 2006;91(9):3451–6.
86. Klingensmith GJ, Garcia SC, Jones HW, et al. Glucocorticoid treatment of girls with congenital adrenal hyperplasia: effects on height, sexual maturation, and fertility. J Pediatr 1977;90(6):996–1004.
87. Grant D, Muram D, Dewhurst J. Menstrual and fertility patterns in patients with congenital adrenal hyperplasia. Pediatr Adolesc Gynecol 1983;1:97–103.
88. Kuhnle U, Bullinger M, Schwarz HP, et al. The quality of life in adult female patients with congenital adrenal hyperplasia: a comprehensive study of the impact of genital malformations and chronic disease on female patients life. Eur J Pediatr 1995;154(9):708–16.
89. Lo JC, Schwitzgebel VM, Tyrrell JB, et al. Normal female infants born of mothers with classic congenital adrenal hyperplasia due to 21-hydroxylase deficiency. J Clin Endocrinol Metab 1999;84(3):930–6.

90. Dumic M, Janjanin N, Ille J, et al. Pregnancy outcomes in women with classical congenital adrenal hyperplasia due to 21-hydroxylase deficiency. J Pediatr Endocrinol Metab 2005;18(9):887–95.

91. Kulshreshtha B, Marumudi E, Khurana ML, et al. Fertility among women with classical congenital adrenal hyperplasia: report of seven cases where treatment was started after 9 years of age. Gynecol Endocrinol 2008;24(5):267–72.

92. Hagenfeldt K, Janson PO, Holmdahl G, et al. Fertility and pregnancy outcome in women with congenital adrenal hyperplasia due to 21-hydroxylase deficiency. Hum Reprod 2008;23(7):1607–13.

93. Yu H, Bian XM, Liu JT, et al. Pregnancy outcomes of eight pregnant women with congenital adrenal hyperplasia due to 21-hydroxylase deficiency. Zhonghua Fu Chan Ke Za Zhi 2012;47(9):651–4.

94. Dörr HG, Hess J, Penger T, et al. Miscarriages in families with an offspring that have classic congenital adrenal hyperplasia and 21-hydroxylase deficiency. BMC Pregnancy and Childbirth 2018;18:456.

95. Hazard J, Guilhaume B, Requeda E, et al. Late diagnosis hyperandrogenism due to adrenal enzyme deficiency (author's transl). Sem Hop 1980;56(47–68): 1975–8.

96. Simm PJ, Zacharin MR. Successful pregnancy in a patient with severe 11-beta-hydroxylase deficiency and novel mutations in CYP11B1 gene. Horm Res 2007; 68(6):294–7.

97. Rabinovici J, Blankstein J, Goldman B, et al. In vitro fertilization and primary embryonic cleavage are possible in 17 alpha-hydroxylase deficiency despite extremely low intrafollicular 17 beta-estradiol. J Clin Endocrinol Metab 1989; 68(3):693–7.

98. Pellicer A, Miró F, Sampaio M, et al. In vitro fertilization as a diagnostic and therapeutic tool in a patient with partial 17,20-desmolase deficiency. Fertil Steril 1991;55(5):970–5.

99. Neuwinger J, Licht P, Munzer B, et al. Substitution with testosterone as aromatizable substrate for induction of follicular maturation, estradiol production and ovulation in a patient with 17 alpha-hydroxylase deficiency. Exp Clin Endocrinol Diabetes 1996;104(5):400–8.

100. Levran D, Ben-Shlomo I, Pariente C, et al. Familial partial 17,20-desmolase and 17alpha-hydroxylase deficiency presenting as infertility. J Assist Reprod Genet 2003;20:21–8.

101. Matsuzaki S, Yanase T, Murakami T, et al. Induction of endometrial cycles and ovulation in a woman with combined 17alpha-hydroxylase/17,20-lyase deficiency due to compound heterozygous mutations on the p45017alpha gene. Fertil Steril 2000;73(6):1183–6.

102. Bianchi PH, Gouveia GR, Costa EM, et al. Successful Live Birth in a Woman With 17α-Hydroxylase Deficiency Through IVF Frozen-Thawed Embryo Transfer. J Clin Endocrinol Metab 2016;101(2):345–8.

103. Kitajima M, Miura K, Inoue T, et al. Two consecutive successful live birth in woman with 17α hydroxylase deficiency by frozen-thaw embryo transfer under hormone replacement endometrium preparation. Gynecol Endocrinol 2018; 34(5):381–4.

104. Khoury K, Barbar E, Ainmelk Y, et al. Gonadal function, first cases of pregnancy, and child delivery in a woman with lipoid congenital adrenal hyperplasia. J Clin Endocrinol Metab 2009;94(4):1333–7.

105. Sertedaki A, Pantos K, Vrettou C, et al. Conception and pregnancy outcome in a patient with 11-bp deletion of the steroidogenic acute regulatory protein gene. Fertil Steril 2009;91(3):934.e15-8.
106. Albarel F, Perrin J, Jegaden M, et al. Successful IVF pregnancy despite inadequate ovarian steroidogenesis due to congenital lipoid adrenal hyperplasia (CLAH): a case report. Hum Reprod 2016;31(11):2609–12.
107. Song T, Wang B, Chen H, et al. In vitro fertilization-frozen embryo transfer in a patient with cytochrome P450 oxidoreductase deficiency: a case report. Gynecol Endocrinol 2018;34(5):385–8.

Calcium Metabolic Disorders in Pregnancy

Primary Hyperparathyroidism, Pregnancy-Induced Osteoporosis, and Vitamin D Deficiency in Pregnancy

Julius Simoni Leere, MD[a,b,*], Peter Vestergaard, MD, PhD, DMSc[b,c]

KEYWORDS

- Pregnancy • Calcium metabolism • Vitamin D • Primary hyperparathyroidism
- Hypoparathyroidism • Osteoporosis

KEY POINTS

- Calcium metabolic disorders are rare in pregnancy and high-quality interventional studies are sparse. Owing to concerns about radiation, radiologic examination of the skeleton is contraindicated throughout pregnancy.
- Primary hyperparathyroidism is mostly asymptomatic and does not seem to affect the ability to conceive or pregnancy outcomes, although complications occur and knowledge on severe cases is missing.
- Primary hyperparathyroidism in pregnancy can mostly be observed with frequent control of plasma calcium levels. In severe cases, surgical intervention may be indicated.
- Osteoporosis in or before pregnancy is rare but usually diagnosed owing to fractures. Medical treatment other than calcium and vitamin D supplementations are generally contraindicated.
- Vitamin D deficiency is common in pregnancy and may affect the chance of conception and risk of complications. Evidence has not proven vitamin D supplementation efficient in improving pregnancy outcomes.

Disclosure Statement: The authors declare they have no conflicts of interest.
Declarations of Interests: None.
[a] Department of Clinical Medicine and Endocrinology, Aalborg University, Aalborg University Hospital, Aalborg, Denmark; [b] Department of Endocrinology, Aalborg University Hospital, Mølleparkvej 4, Aalborg 9000, Denmark; [c] Steno Diabetes Center North Jutland, Aalborg, Denmark
* Corresponding author. Department of Endocrinology, Aalborg University Hospital, Mølleparkvej 4, Aalborg 9000, Denmark.
E-mail address: j.leere@rn.dk

INTRODUCTION
General Considerations

Most calcium metabolic disorders are rare in pregnancy and thus most studies are observational with few high-quality interventional studies except for vitamin D supplementation, for which randomized controlled trials have been performed.[1] The following is a short description of the current evidence on the most common conditions.

Physiology

During pregnancy many physiologic changes occur, including changes in calcium and phosphate, and calciotropic hormone status.[1,2]

During the pregnancy, the placenta and, later, the lactating mammary glands, produce parathyroid hormone–related peptide (PTHrP), which, among other things, has effects similar to parathyroid hormone except for a slightly different effect on the parathyroid hormone 2 receptor (**Fig. 1**).[1] The placenta may also be involved in vitamin D production.[3]

PTHrP tends to mobilize calcium from the skeleton through osteoclast-induced resorption and thus maintain calcium levels despite increased consumption for the fetus and, later, through the breast milk to the newborn child.[1]

Owing to concerns about radiation, regular radiographic examinations and radiation-based examinations, such as dual-energy X-ray absorptiometry (DEXA), cannot be performed during pregnancy except for in the forearm, with proper radiation protection of the mother and fetus.

Methods

A systematic literature search of Medline was performed for all topics covered. Emphasis was placed on clinical studies; that is, observational or interventional studies on pregnant or lactating women, as well as women trying to conceive.

PRIMARY HYPERPARATHYROIDISM

A search of Medline on June 2, 2018, using the terms "primary hyperparathyroidism" (PHPT) and "pregnancy" resulted in 223 papers.

Incidence

Pregnancy and delivery among women with PHPT is rare because PHPT is usually seen among women outside potential childbearing age.[4] In a population study by Abood and Vestergaard,[5] based on the Danish National Registers for diagnostic codes, covering 1977 to 2010 (both years included), 262 live births were registered before the diagnosis of PHPT was made and 1273 after. In the same period, 2,114,960 live births were recorded in the background population.[6] This yields a rate of 72.6 (95% CI 69.0–76.3) births among patients ever diagnosed with PHPT per 100,000 live births. Among these 1535 live births, 380, with a rate of 18.0 (95% CI 16.2–19.9) per 100,000, took place between 1 and 5 years before the year the diagnosis was made, with the births likely taking place in women with active PHPT. Within 1 year following the diagnosis, the number of live births was 70, yielding a rate of 3.3 (95% CI 2.6–4.2) per 100,000 in women with a known diagnosis of active PHPT. This is compatible with what was seen in the North Denmark Region from 2012 to 2017 (both years included), where 2 pregnancies with live births (no abortions and no stillbirths) among women with PHPT were observed among 33,410 live births, with a rate of 6.0 (95% CI 1.6–21.8) per 100,000 women per year (P. Vestergaard, personal

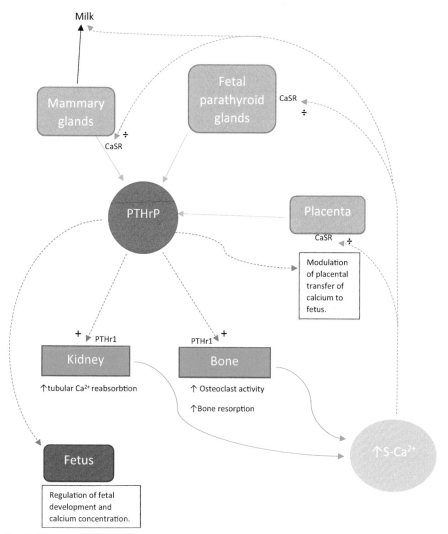

Fig. 1. Humoral effects of PTHrP during pregnancy. PTHrP is secreted during pregnancy and lactation from the placenta, mammary glands, and the fetal parathyroid glands. In kidney and bone, increased calcium reabsorption and bone resorption leads to an increased availability of calcium in the blood for fetal development and, later, milk production. The secretion is regulated by negative feedback via the calcium-sensing receptor (CaSR). Ca^{2+}, Calcium ion; $S-Ca^{2+}$, Serum Calcium.

communication, 2019). A study by DiMarco and colleagues[7] reported an expected incidence of 0.05% (50/100.000) during pregnancy, whereas other studies have reported a frequency as high as 0.5% to 1.4%.[8] However, as previously outlined, these numbers may be rather high compared with population experience.

Clinical Consequences of Primary Hyperparathyroidism Before, During, and After Pregnancy

Ability to conceive

Few studies exist concerning the ability to conceive. A large population-based study by Abood and Vestergaard[5] based on 1057 women of childbearing age with PHPT found that the number of pregnancies, abortions, live births, and the outcome of live births (Apgar score, length, and weight of the newborn) did not differ from that of an age-matched and gender-matched control group, even within the last year before the diagnosis. It may thus seem that the ability to conceive and pregnancy outcome in general are not affected in PHPT, although knowledge regarding women with severe cases is lacking.

Live births and complications

Abood and Vestergaard[5] reported that, following the PHPT diagnosis, the number of women giving birth did not differ between the 2 groups. Birthweight, birth length, Apgar score, and gestation length at birth did not differ. Within the first year after the diagnosis was made, gestation length was lower in women with PHPT than in controls. However, this was linked to more deliveries by cesarean sections, which were probably caused by a clinical desire to terminate the pregnancy early, possibly to allow diagnostic evaluation with sestamibi scintigraphy and subsequent neck surgery.

A study by Hirsch and colleagues[9] reported no difference in obstetric complications among women with PHPT. The favorable prognosis for pregnancy and delivery in PHPT has furthermore been supported by a small case series.[10]

Abortions

The study by Abood and Vestergaard[5] reported no excess of abortions following PHPT diagnosis and before the diagnosis was made, even within the last year before diagnosis. This was confirmed by Hirsch and colleagues,[9] who similarly reported no difference in abortions.

DiMarco and colleagues[7] reported 1 case of PHPT diagnosed among 289 women with recurrent miscarriages (0.34%), reporting that this was higher than the 0.05% expected. However, a post hoc calculation yielded a likelihood of 0.34% (95% CI 0.06%–1.93%), which was not far from what was expected. Because the uncertainty is large, this finding must be taken with caution, particularly when keeping in mind the frequency of PHPT in pregnancies reported elsewhere.[8]

In contrast to the previously mentioned studies, Norman and colleagues[11] reported that PHPT is associated with a 3.5-fold increase in miscarriage rates. Pregnancy loss often occurred in the second trimester and was associated with multiple miscarriages when not addressed. Pregnancy loss was more common because calcium levels exceeded 11.4 mg/dL (2.85 mmol/L), but this may be seen at all elevated calcium levels. The study by Norman and colleagues[11] was based on 77 pregnancies in 32 subjects from a single center (0.7% of all PHPT cases in the center's total cohort) and may perhaps represent selected cases, although the observation from more severe cases warrants consideration.

In case of a history of recurrent pregnancy loss, surgical intervention may perhaps be considered, although there is no evidence to support this.[12]

Clinical Considerations

Complications

PHPT is often asymptomatic and mild[13] especially in pregnancy,[9] although complications may span from hypercalcemic crisis (women with hyperemesis being prone to this owing to dehydration) due to symptomatic urinary tract stones (although most calcifications are asymptomatic),[14] acute pancreatitis,[15] depression, cardiovascular events, and gastric and duodenal ulcers.

Differential diagnoses

PHPT is primarily seen among women.[16,17] The differential diagnosis is familial (benign) hypocalciuric hypercalcemia,[18] which requires no intervention except for acute surgical intervention in the rare case that the child is born with neonatal severe hyperparathyroidism[19] due to homozygous inactivation of the calcium-sensing receptor (CaSR).[20] In rare cases, parathyroid carcinomas may be encountered.[21] In these cases, CDC73 mutations should be suspected.[22]

Because women of potential childbearing are younger than patients usually diagnosed with PHPT,[4] the proportion with genetically linked multiple endocrine neoplasia (MEN)-1 and MEN2[23] may be higher, as are the proportion with familial PHPT (CDC73 mutations), than seen among older women with PHPT.

Management

The only curative treatment in symptomatic women is surgical intervention.[24] Sestamibi scintigraphy has been used in selected cases[25] but may be avoided owing to the use of radionuclides,[24] leaving ultrasonography of the neck as the only diagnostic location available, provided that focused operation rather than bilateral neck exploration should be performed.[26] In general, management with observation and sufficient fluid intake may be the preferred choice in most cases.

General anesthesia, as well as focused surgery with local analgesia,[27] may be used, depending on the situation, if surgical intervention is needed. In experienced hands, surgical management seems safe in pregnant women.[5] The risks are those of surgical management of PHPT in general; that is, hypoparathyroidism, recurrent laryngeal nerve paralysis, bleeding, infection, and postoperative pain.

Cinacalcet[28] and calcitonin may be used as medical management in selected cases of symptomatic hypercalcemia during pregnancy, but these require further investigation. Bisphosphonates should be restricted to life-threatening hypercalcemia.[24]

In case of vitamin D deficiency, vitamin D may be supplemented. Calcium supplements should be discontinued.

The main consideration for the neonate is the risk of hypocalcemia due to suppression of the fetal parathyroid glands.[12]

Summary

PHPT in pregnancy may be observed with control of plasma calcium levels and encouragement of adequate fluid intake. In case of very high and increasing calcium levels, and in symptomatic cases, surgical intervention may be indicated. When surgery is indicated, it may preferably be performed in the second trimester if possible.[12]

HYPOPARATHYROIDISM

A systematic search of Medline on June 2, 2018, resulted in 381 papers.

Hypoparathyroidism in pregnant women is primarily a complication from neck surgery performed before or during pregnancy, although autoimmune disease and rare cases of hereditary disorders do occur.[29]

Little is known about the ability to conceive; pregnancy outcomes, such as abortion risk; and the outcome of live births, such as Apgar score, birthweight, and birth length.[30,31]

In patients with preexisting hypoparathyroidism, the need for supplementation with calcium and vitamin D may increase,[32,33] although a decreased need for supplementation with activated vitamin D and calcium may be seen during pregnancy and lactation.[34] The latter is probably due to PTHrP production in the placenta intrapartum and, later, in the breast during lactation.[35]

The calcium levels thus require close monitoring during and immediately following delivery and during lactation owing to the risk of hypercalcemia, hypocalcemia, and milk-alkali syndrome.[36]

The neonate may experience hypercalcemia from intoxication of the mother with calcium and activated vitamin D, as well as hypocalcemia from insufficient substitution.[37]

If the cause of hypoparathyroidism is not surgical but due to inherited syndromes, these may be transferred to the newborn.

Autosomal dominant hypocalcemia due to activating mutations in the CaSR may require no treatment with activated vitamin D and calcium owing to the risk of renal calcifications.[38]

Summary

Hypoparathyroidism in pregnancy is uncommon. Management is based on supplementations and close monitoring of plasma(p)-calcium and p-vitamin D levels.

OSTEOPOROSIS

A search of PubMed on June 2, 2018 resulted in 1102 publications.

Epidemiology and Pathophysiology

Osteoporosis is rare in young women[39] and may be related to other conditions, such as hyperthyroidism and treatment with glucocorticoids.[40] Thus osteoporosis in and before pregnancy is rare. Young women rarely undergo screening for osteoporosis with DEXA, and, therefore, the diagnosis in and before pregnancy is usually due to fractures; that is, symptomatic osteoporosis.[2]

In patients with secondary osteoporosis or primary osteoporosis, the cause may be related to PTHrP from placenta during pregnancy and breast during lactation, causing increased bone resorption, leading to fractures, especially of the spine.[2] Pregnancy-associated transient osteoporosis of the hip is rare and characterized by lowered bone mineral density (BMD) in the femoral head and neck, and simultaneous hip pain late in pregnancy. It is vaguely described in the literature and its cause is not fully understood.[41,42]

Several factors affecting bone metabolism, such as estrogens or prolactin, are elevated during pregnancy; however, their effect is not clear.[2] An increase in the ratio of receptor activator of nuclear factor kappa-β ligand (RANKL) to osteoprotegerin increases bone resorption, which may lead to osteoporosis and fragility fracture.[2] The condition is transitory, and long-term studies do not link the number of pregnancies with osteoporosis.[2]

Osteoporosis in 1 pregnancy may thus not predict recurrence in subsequent pregnancies.

Clinical Consequences

During pregnancy and lactation, BMD may decrease.[43] Kolthoff and colleagues[43] followed 59 women during pregnancy and lactation and reported a differential pattern of changes in bone density at different skeletal sites. The reduction in the ultradistal radius during pregnancy amounted to 2% with no further changes during lactation. After delivery, the reduction in BMD was most pronounced in the spine (5.2% in 3 months), but the decline in bone mass tended to revert after resumption of menstruation. BMD remained reduced by 3.3% after 12 months in women with menstruation resumption later than 8 months after delivery. No significant reduction was observed

18 months after delivery. No association with calcium intake, weight changes, or initial BMD was observed. High calcium intake did not protect against bone mineral loss in the spine and the femur. Thus, it can be concluded that bone loss during pregnancy and lactation took place mainly from the trabecular skeleton. Resumption of menstruation tended to result in a regain of bone mass toward baseline.[43]

Management

The treatment is calcium and vitamin D. The safety of several antiosteoporotic drugs during pregnancy is uncertain. Bisphosphonates administered during pregnancy or released from bone treated prophylactically before pregnancy may cross the placenta and interact with fetal bone formation. Use in pregnancy should be carefully balanced against risks.[44] Several case studies on mothers receiving various bisphosphonates, mainly for secondary osteoporosis, before or throughout pregnancy report no adverse events in either mother or child, but evidence is weak.[45–47] Bisphosphonates can be resumed after delivery and lactation. Raloxifene is not indicated in premenopausal women; that is, women with childbearing potential.[48] Teriparatide should not be used with open epiphyseal lines and is, therefore, not indicated in pregnant women owing to the potential fetal harm.[49] Denosumab is contraindicated in pregnant women owing to potential fetal harm.[50] Case reports have described the use of calcitonin, bisphosphonates, strontium ranelate, teriparatide, vertebroplasty, and kyphoplasty to treat postpartum vertebral fractures. However, the need for such treatments is uncertain given that a progressive increase in bone mass subsequently occurs in most women who present with a fracture during pregnancy or lactation.[51]

Pain from spine fractures may be treated by bed rest and analgesics along usual guidelines in women. In case of immobilization, prophylaxis against venous thromboembolism may be considered. After delivery, antiosteoporotic drugs may be resumed if the criteria for their use are met.

Lactation may be discouraged because this accelerates bone loss.[2]

Calcium and vitamin D may be continued during pregnancy.

Summary

Osteoporosis is rare and often secondary to other comorbidities in pregnancy. BMD is reduced during pregnancy and lactation but reverts after resumption of menstruation. Treatment should be limited to calcium and vitamin D supplementation whenever possible, and antiresorptive therapy should be paused until after delivery and lactation unless there is absolute indication.

VITAMIN D DEFICIENCY AND SUPPLEMENTATION

A search of PubMed June 2, 2018 with the search words "vitamin D" and "pregnancy" resulted in 3836 articles. Limiting the search to clinical trials resulted in 170 articles.

Vitamin D deficiency is common worldwide[52] and thus also among pregnant and lactating women.[53]

Improved vitamin D status may be associated with better chance of conception.[54]

Children born preterm may have low vitamin D levels, which may increase after supplementation.[55,56] Supplementation with vitamin D in lactating women may also increase breast milk and infant vitamin D status.[57,58]

High vitamin D levels may be associated with lower risk of preeclampsia, but vitamin D supplementation did not reduce this risk,[59] although calcium plus vitamin D improved blood pressure and other metabolic markers.[60]

In nonindustrialized countries, vitamin D supplementation may reduce the combined endpoint of preterm labor, preeclampsia, or gestational diabetes and may be associated with higher birthweight.[61]

One study controversially reported an increased risk of gestational diabetes with rising vitamin D levels in a Hispanic subgroup,[62] but this association has not been reproduced in other cohorts, and the opposite has been seen in other studies.[63] Improved pregnancy outcomes have even been seen with supplementation in women with gestational diabetes.[64]

Some studies have reported on nonclinical endpoints.[65,66]

Low vitamin D levels may be associated with a decreased likelihood of live birth.[67] However, studies on clinical endpoints have failed to report improvements in offspring outcomes,[68] including bone measures in women and offspring,[69,70] and health care utilization.[71]

High-dose vitamin D supplementation has not been shown to increase BMD in pregnant women.[72,73]

Low vitamin D levels may be associated with an increased risk of perinatal depression.[74] One study reported decreased risk of perinatal depression with vitamin D supplementation.[75]

Vitamin D supplementation may decrease the likelihood of allergen sensitization,[76] and the risk of wheezing may also be reduced.[77,78]

A meta-analysis concluded that vitamin D supplementation during pregnancy was associated with increased circulating 25-Vitamin D levels, birthweight, and birth length, and was not associated with other maternal and neonatal outcomes. In contrast, incidence of preeclampsia, GDM, small for gestational age, low birthweight, preterm birth, and cesarean section were not influenced by vitamin D supplementation.[79]

Summary

Vitamin D supplementation may, in general, not improve pregnancy outcomes.

RARE DISEASES

Little evidence on rare diseases is present. The following is from the clinical impression.

Osteogenesis imperfecta: The child may inherit the condition, and the mother may risk spine fractures from carrying the child.

Hypophosphatemic rickets: Usually the pregnancy is uneventful, and the child may inherit the condition. Doses of supplements with activated vitamin D may have to be changed along the lines of pregnant women with hypoparathyroidism.

Pseudohypoparathyroidism: This is usually uneventful.

REFERENCES

1. Thomsen S vid S. Vitamin D status in the first 9 months of life. 2011;I. https://doi.org/10.15713/ins.mmj.3.

2. Sanz-Salvador L, Garcia-Perez MA, Tarin JJ, et al. Bone metabolic changes during pregnancy: a period of vulnerability to osteoporosis and fracture. Eur J Endocrinol 2015;172(2):R53–65.

3. Park H, Wood MR, Malysheva OV, et al. Placental vitamin D metabolism and its associations with circulating vitamin D metabolites in pregnant women. Am J Clin Nutr 2017;106(6):1439–48.

4. Abood A, Vestergaard P. Increasing incidence of primary hyperparathyroidism in Denmark. Dan Med J 2013;60:1–5.
5. Abood A, Vestergaard P. Pregnancy outcomes in women with primary hyperparathyroidism. Eur J Endocrinol 2014;171(1):69–76.
6. Statistikbanken. Available at: www.statistikbanken.dk. Accessed February 1, 2019.
7. DiMarco A, Christakis I, Constantinides V, et al. Undiagnosed primary hyperparathyroidism and recurrent miscarriage: the first prospective pilot study. World J Surg 2018;42(3):639–45.
8. Komarowska H, Bromińska B, Luftmann B, et al. Primary hyperparathyroidism in pregnan–y - a review of literature. Ginekol Pol 2017;88(5):270–5.
9. Hirsch D, Kopel V, Nadler V, et al. Pregnancy outcomes in women with primary hyperparathyroidism. J Clin Endocrinol Metab 2015;100(5):2115–22.
10. Rchachi M, El Ouahabi H, Boujraf S, et al. Primary hyperparathyroidism in pregnancy. Ann Afr Med 2017;16(3):145–7.
11. Norman J, Politz D, Politz L. Hyperparathyroidism during pregnancy and the effect of rising calcium on pregnancy loss: a call for earlier intervention. Clin Endocrinol (Oxf) 2009;71(1):104–9.
12. Diaz-Soto G, Linglart A, Senat M-V-, et al. Primary hyperparathyroidism in pregnancy. Endocrine 2013;44(3):591–7. Available at: http://ovidsp.ovid.com/ovidweb.cgi?T=JS&PAGE=reference&D=emed15&NEWS=N&AN=52580286.
13. Leere JS, Karmisholt J, Robaczyk M, et al. Contemporary medical management of primary hyperparathyroidism: a systematic review. Front Endocrinol (Lausanne) 2017;8:1–11.
14. Starup-Linde J, Waldhauer E, Rolighed L, et al. Renal stones and calcifications in patients with primary hyperparathyroidism: associations with biochemical variables. Eur J Endocrinol 2012;166(6):1093–100.
15. Han ES, Fritton K, Bacon P, et al. Preterm parturient with polyhydramnios and pancreatitis: primary presentation of hyperparathyroidism. Case Rep Obstet Gynecol 2018;2018:2091082.
16. Vestergaard P, Mollerup CL, Frokjaer VG, et al. Cohort study of risk of fracture before and after surgery for primary hyperparathyroidism. BMJ 2000; 321(7261):598–602. Available at: http://www.ncbi.nlm.nih.gov/pubmed/10977834.
17. Vestergaard P, Mosekilde L. Cohort study on effects of parathyroid surgery on multiple outcomes in primary hyperparathyroidism. BMJ 2003;327(7414):530–4.
18. Christensen SE, Nissen PH, Vestergaard P, et al. Familial hypocalciuric hypercalcaemia: a review. Curr Opin Endocrinol Diabetes Obes 2011;18(6):359–70.
19. Maltese G, Izatt L, Mcgowan BM, et al. Making (mis) sense of asymptomatic marked hypercalcemia in pregnancy. Key Clinical Message. Clin Case Rep 2017;1587–90.
20. Gannon AW, Monk HM, Levine MA. Cinacalcet monotherapy in neonatal severe hyperparathyroidism: a case study and review. J Clin Endocrinol Metab 2014; 99(1):7–11.
21. Paul RG, Elston MS, Gill AJ, et al. Hypercalcaemia due to parathyroid carcinoma presenting in the third trimester of pregnancy. Aust N Z J Obstet Gynaecol 2012; 52(2):204–7.
22. Gill AJ, Lim G, Cheung VKY, et al. Parafibromin-deficient (HPT-JT type, CDC73 mutated) parathyroid tumors demonstrate distinctive morphologic features. Am J Surg Pathol 2019. https://doi.org/10.1097/PAS.0000000000001017.

23. Nagamura Y, Yamazaki M, Shimazu S, et al. A novel splice site mutation of the MEN1 gene identified in a patient with primary hyperparathyroidism. Endocr J 2012;59(6):523–30.
24. Dochez V, Ducarme G. Primary hyperparathyroidism during pregnancy. Arch Gynecol Obstet 2015;291(2):259–63. Available at: http://ovidsp.ovid.com/ovidweb. cgi?T=JS&PAGE=reference&D=medl&NEWS=N&AN=25367603.
25. Rubin MR, Silverberg SJ. Use of cinacalcet and 99mtc-sestamibi imaging during pregnancy. J Endocr Soc 2017;1(9):1156–9.
26. Hu Y, Cui M, Sun Z, et al. Clinical presentation, management, and outcomes of primary hyperparathyroidism during pregnancy. Int J Endocrinol 2017;2017. https://doi.org/10.1155/2017/3947423.
27. Zeng H, Li Z, Zhang X, et al. Anesthetic management of primary hyperparathyroidism during pregnancy. Medicine (Baltimore) 2017;96(51):e9390.
28. Gonzalo García I, Robles Fradejas M, Martín Macías M de los A, et al. Primary hyperparathyroidism in pregnancy treated with cinacalcet: a case report. J Obstet Gynaecol 2018;38(1):132–4.
29. Lopes MP, Kliemann BS, Bini IB, et al. Hypoparathyroidism and pseudohypoparathyroidism: etiology, laboratory features and complications. Arch Endocrinol Metab 2016;60(6):532–6.
30. Arredondo F, Noble L. Endocrinology of recurrent pregnancy loss. Semin Reprod Med 2006;24(1):33–9.
31. Kohlmeier L, Marcus R. Calcium disorders of pregnancy. Endocrinol Metab Clin North Am 1995;24(1):15–39.
32. Callies F, Arlt W, Scholz HJ, et al. Management of hypoparathyroidism during pregna–y–report of twelve cases. Eur J Endocrinol 1998;139(3):284–9.
33. Shah KH, Bhat S, Shetty S, et al. Hypoparathyroidism in pregnancy. BMJ Case Rep 2015. https://doi.org/10.1136/bcr-2015-210228. bcr2015210228.
34. Dixon J, Miller S. Successful pregnancies and reduced treatment requirement while breast feeding in a patient with congenital hypoparathyroidism due to homozygous c.68C>A null parathyroid hormone gene mutation. BMJ Case Rep 2018. https://doi.org/10.1136/bcr-2017-223811.
35. Mestman J. Parathyroid disorders of pregnancy. Semin Perinatol 1998;22(6):485–96.
36. Skwarek A, Pachucki J, Bednarczuk T, et al. Milk-alkali syndrome (MAS) as a complication of the treatment of hypoparathyroidi–m - a case study. Endokrynol Pol 2018;69(2):200–4.
37. Demirel N, Aydin M, Zenciroglu A, et al. Hyperparathyroidism secondary to maternal hypoparathyroidism and vitamin D deficiency: an uncommon cause of neonatal respiratory distress. Ann Trop Paediatr 2009;29(2):149–54.
38. Mayr B, Schnabel D, Dörr H-G, et al. GENETICS IN ENDOCRINOLOGY: gain and loss of function mutations of the calcium-sensing receptor and associated proteins: current treatment concepts. Eur J Endocrinol 2016;174(5):R189–208.
39. Vestergaard P, Rejnmark L, Mosekilde L. Osteoporosis is markedly underdiagnosed: a nationwide study from Denmark. Osteoporos Int 2005;16(2):134–41.
40. Vestergaard P, Rejnmark L, Mosekilde L. Fracture risk associated with systemic and topical corticosteroids. J Intern Med 2005;257:374–84.
41. Hadji P, Boekhoff J, Hahn M, et al. Pregnancy-associated transient osteoporosis of the hip: results of a case-control study. Arch Osteoporos 2017;12(1). https://doi.org/10.1007/s11657-017-0310-y.
42. Kovacs CS. Calcium and bone metabolism in pregnancy and lactation. J Clin Endocrinol Metab 2001;86(6):2344–8.

43. Kolthoff N, Eiken P, Kristensen B, et al. Bone mineral changes during pregnancy and lactation: a longitudinal cohort study. Clin Sci 1998;94(4):405–12.
44. rxlist.com. rxlist.com – tilizamax precautions. Available at: https://www.rxlist.com/fosamax-drug.htm#warnings_precautions. Accessed February 1, 2019.
45. Ioannis SP, Chrysoula LG, Aikaterini K, et al. The use of bisphosphonates in women prior to or during pregnancy and lactation. Hormones 2011;10(4):280–91.
46. Djokanovic N, Klieger-Grossmann C, Koren G. Does treatment with bisphosphonates endanger the human pregnancy? J Obstet Gynaecol Can 2008;30(12): 1146–8.
47. Vujasinovic-Stupar N, Pejnovic N, Markovic L, et al. Pregnancy-associated spinal osteoporosis treated with bisphosphonates: long-term follow-up of maternal and infants outcome. Rheumatol Int 2012;32(3):819–23.
48. rxlist.com. rxlist.com - Raloxifene precautions. Available at: https://www.rxlist.com/evista-drug.htm#description. Accessed February 1, 2019.
49. rxlist.com. rxlist.com - Forteo precautions. Available at: https://www.rxlist.com/forteo-drug.htm. Accessed February 1, 2019.
50. rxlist.com. rxlist.com - Prolia precautions. Available at: https://www.rxlist.com/prolia-drug.htm#warnings_precautions. Accessed February 1, 2019.
51. Kovacs CS, Ralston SH. Presentation and management of osteoporosis presenting in association with pregnancy or lactation. Osteoporos Int 2015;26(9): 2223–41.
52. Hagenau T, Vest R, Gissel TN, et al. Global vitamin D levels in relation to age, gender, skin pigmentation and latitude: an ecologic meta-regression analysis. Osteoporos Int 2009;20(1):133–40.
53. Xiao J-P, Zang J, Pei J-J, et al. Low maternal vitamin D status during the second trimester of pregnancy: a cross-sectional study in Wuxi, China. PLoS One 2015; 10(2):e0117748.
54. Lerchbaum E, Rabe T. Vitamin D and female fertility. Curr Opin Obstet Gynecol 2014;26(3):145–50.
55. Anderson-Berry A, Thoene M, Wagner J, et al. Randomized trial of two doses of vitamin D3 in preterm infants. PLoS One 2017;12(10):e0185950.
56. Rodda CP, Benson JE, Vincent AJ, et al. Maternal Vitamin D supplementation during pregnancy prevents Vitamin D deficiency in the newborn: an open-label randomized controlled trial. Clin Endocrinol (Oxf) 2015;83(3):363–8.
57. Wall CR, Stewart AW, Camargo C Jr, et al. Vitamin D activity of breast milk in women randomly assigned to vitamin D3 supplementation during pregnancy. Am J Clin Nutr 2016;103(2):382–8.
58. March KM, Chen NN, Karakochuk CD, et al. Erratum for March et al. Maternal vitamin D3 supplementation at 50 µg/d protects against low serum 25-hydroxyvitamin D in infants at 8 wk of age: a randomized controlled trial of 3 doses of vitamin D beginning in gestation and continued in lactation. Am J Clin Nutr 2016;104(5):1491.
59. Mirzakhani H, Litonjua AA, McElrath TF, et al. Early pregnancy vitamin D status and risk of preeclampsia. J Clin Invest 2016;126(12). https://doi.org/10.1172/JCI89031DS1.
60. Samimi M, Kashi M, Foroozanfard F, et al. The effects of vitamin D plus calcium supplementation on metabolic profiles, biomarkers of inflammation, oxidative stress and pregnancy outcomes in pregnant women at risk for pre-eclampsia. J Hum Nutr Diet 2016;29(4):505–15.

61. Sablok A, Batra A, Thariani K, et al. Supplementation of Vitamin D in pregnancy and its correlation with feto-maternal outcome. Clin Endocrinol (Oxf) 2015;83(4): 536–41.

62. Nobles CJ, Markenson G, Chasan-Taber L. Early pregnancy Vitamin D status and risk for adverse maternal and infant outcomes in a bi-ethnic cohort: the behaviors affecting baby and you (B.A.B.Y.) Study. Br J Nutr 2015;114(12):2116–28.

63. Karamali M, Beihaghi E, Mohammadi A, et al. Effects of high-dose vitamin D supplementation on metabolic status and pregnancy outcomes in pregnant women at risk for pre-eclampsia. Horm Metab Res 2015;47(12):867–72.

64. Karamali M, Asemi Z, Ahmadi-Dastjerdi M, et al. Calcium plus Vitamin D supplementation affects pregnancy outcomes in gestational diabetes: randomized, double-blind, placebo-controlled trial. Public Health Nutr 2016;19(1):156–63.

65. Zerofsky MS, Jacoby BN, Pedersen TL, et al. Daily cholecalciferol supplementation during pregnancy alters markers of regulatory immunity, inflammation, and clinical outcomes in a randomized controlled trial. J Nutr 2016;146(11):2388–97.

66. Sordillo JE, Zhou Y, McGeachie MJ, et al. Factors influencing the infant gut microbiome at age 3-6 months: findings from the ethnically diverse Vitamin D Antenatal Asthma Reduction Trial (VDAART). J Allergy Clin Immunol 2017;139(2): 482–91.e14.

67. Pal L, Zhang H, Williams J, et al. Vitamin D status relates to reproductive outcome in women with polycystic ovary syndrome: secondary analysis of a multicenter randomized controlled trial. J Clin Endocrinol Metab 2016;101(8):3027–35.

68. Sahoo SK, Katam KK, Das V, et al. Maternal vitamin D supplementation in pregnancy and offspring outcomes: a double-blind randomized placebo-controlled trial. J Bone Miner Metab 2017;35(4):464–71.

69. Vaziri F, Dabbaghmanesh MH, Samsami A, et al. Vitamin D supplementation during pregnancy on infant anthropometric measurements and bone mass of mother-infant pairs: a randomized placebo clinical trial. Early Hum Dev 2016; 103(2016):61–8.

70. Cooper C, Harvey NC, Bishop NJ, et al. Maternal gestational vitamin D supplementation and offspring bone health (MAVIDOS): a multicentre, double-blind, randomised placebo-controlled trial. Lancet Diabetes Endocrinol 2016;4(5): 393–402.

71. Griffiths M, Goldring S, Griffiths C, et al. Effects of pre-Natal Vitamin D supplementation with partial correction of Vitamin D deficiency on early life healthcatilizationion: a randomised controlled trial. PLoS One 2015;10(12):1–19.

72. Wei W, Shary J, Garrett-Mayer E, et al. Bone mineral density during pregnancy in women participating in a randomized controlled trial of vitamin D supplementation. Am J Clin Nutr 2017;106(6):1422–30.

73. Diogenes MEL, Bezerra FF, Rezende EP, et al. Calcium plus vitamin D supplementation during the third trimester of pregnancy in adolescents accustomed to low calcium diets does not affect infant bone mass at early lactation in a randomized controlled trial. J Nutr 2015;145(7):1515–23.

74. Williams JA, Romero VC, Clinton CM, et al. Vitamin D levels and perinatal depressive symptoms in women at risk: a secondary analysis of the mothers, omega-3, and mental health study. BMC Pregnancy Childbirth 2016;16(1):1–9.

75. Vaziri F, Nasiri S, Tavana Z, et al. A randomized controlled trial of vitamin D supplementation on perinatal depression: in Iranian pregnant mothers. BMC Pregnancy Childbirth 2016;16(1):1–12.

76. Grant CC, Crane J, Mitchell EA, et al. Vitamin D supplementation during pregnancy and infancy reduces aeroallergen sensitization: a randomized controlled trial. Allergy 2016;71(9):1325–34.
77. Chawes BL, Bønnelykke K, Stokholm J, et al. Effect of vitamin D $_3$ supplementation during pregnancy on risk of persistent wheeze in the offspring. JAMA 2016; 315(4):353.
78. Litonjua AA, Carey VJ, Laranjo N, et al. Effect of prenatal supplementation with Vitamin D on asthma or recurrent wheezing in offspring by age 3 years: the VDAART randomized clinical trial. JAMA 2016;315(4):362–70.
79. Pérez-López FR, Pasupuleti V, Mezones-Holguin E, et al. Effect of vitamin D supplementation during pregnancy on maternal and neonatal outcomes: a systematic review and meta-analysis of randomized controlled trials. Fertil Steril 2015; 103(5):1278–88.e4.

Moving?

Make sure your subscription moves with you!

To notify us of your new address, find your **Clinics Account Number** (located on your mailing label above your name), and contact customer service at:

Email: journalscustomerservice-usa@elsevier.com

800-654-2452 (subscribers in the U.S. & Canada)
314-447-8871 (subscribers outside of the U.S. & Canada)

Fax number: 314-447-8029

Elsevier Health Sciences Division
Subscription Customer Service
3251 Riverport Lane
Maryland Heights, MO 63043

*To ensure uninterrupted delivery of your subscription, please notify us at least 4 weeks in advance of move.

Printed and bound by CPI Group (UK) Ltd, Croydon, CR0 4YY

08/05/2025

01864746-0006